Diagnosis in color

Skin Signs in Clinical Medicine

D0933334

Diagnosis in color

Skin Signs in Clinical Medicine

J A Savin
MA MD FRCP DIH

Consultant Dermatologist
University of Edinburgh
Department of Dermatology
The Royal Infirmary of Edinburgh
Edinburgh

J A A Hunter
BA MD FRCPE

Professor of Dermatology
University of Edinburgh
Department of Dermatology
The Royal Infirmary of Edinburgh
Edinburgh

N C Hepburn
MD MRCP

Consultant Dermatologist
Royal Army Medical Corps
Ministry of Defence
London

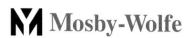 Mosby-Wolfe

London • Baltimore • Barcelona • Bogotá • Boston
Buenos Aires • Carlsbad, CA • Chicago • Madrid
Mexico City • Milan • Naples, FL • New York
Philadelphia • St. Louis • Seoul • Singapore
Sydney • Taipei • Tokyo • Toronto • Wiesbaden

To Patricia, Ruth and Julia - with love

Publisher:	**Richard Furn**
Development Editor:	**Jennifer Prast**
Project Manager:	**Sarah Gray**
Production:	**Jane Tozer**
Index:	**Jill Halliday**
Cover Design:	**Greg Smith**

Copyright © 1997 Times Mirror International Publishers Limited

Published in 1997 by Mosby-Wolfe, an imprint of Times Mirror International Publishers Limited

Printed in Italy by Vincenzo Bona s.r.l., Turin

ISBN 0 7234 2240 0

For full details of all Times Mirror International Publishers Limited titles, please write to Times Mirror International Publishers Limited, Lynton House, 7–12 Tavistock Square, London WC1H 9LB, England.

A CIP catalogue record for this book is available from the British Library.

Contents

Acknowledgements

The clinical photographs come from our departmental collections and we wish to thank all those who presented these. Those given by individuals are listed below:

Dr P. K. Buxton, Department of Dermatology, Royal Infirmary, Edinburgh: 1.6, 1.12, 1.15, 1.17, 1.20 1.23, 1.29, 1.36, 1.41, 1.42, 1.56, 2.20, 2.35, 2.39, 2.45, 3.3, 4.22, 4.26, 4.50, 4.52, 4.55, 4.57, 4.59, 4.74, 4.83, 5.29, 5.51, 6.5, 7.4, 7.5, 7.15, 7.33, 8.42, 9.15, 9.16, 10.9.

Dr E. C. Benton, Department of Dermatology, Royal Infirmary, Edinburgh: 1.103, 4.60, 5.17, 9.12, 10.7.

Dr M. J. Tidman, Department of Dermatology, Royal Infirmary, Edinburgh: 3.14, 7.39, 8.26.

Dr. G. W. Beveridge, Department of Dermatology, Royal Infirmary, Edinburgh: 8.27, 10.5.

Dr H. Horn, Department of Dermatology, Royal Infirmary, Edinburgh: 4.17.

Dr P. D. Welsby, Infectious Diseases Unit, City Hospital, Edinburgh: 1.9, 1.40.

Dr R. S. Bartholomew, Ophthalmology Unit, Royal Infirmary, Edinburgh: 4.30, 4.31.

Dr A. McMillan, Genito-Urinary Medicine Unit, Royal Infirmary, Edinburgh: 1.73, 3.11, 4.38, 4.79, 4.86.

Dr A. D. Toft, Department of Medicine, Royal Infirmary, Edinburgh: 7.14.

Mr J. D. Watson, Plastic Surgery Unit, St John's Hospital, Livingstone: 1.95.

Dr J. G. Lowe, Department of Dermatology, Ninewells Hospital, Dundee: 3.9.

Dr R. I. MacLeod, Dental Hospital, Royal Infirmary, Edinburgh: 4.33, 4.39, 4.40.

Figures 1.32, 1.44, 1.73, 1.116, 2.15, 2.44, 3.11, 3.13, 4.42, 4.49, 4.56, 4.71, 5.8, 5.28, 5.39, 7.1, 7.29, 7.30, 8.37, 8.45 and 10.2 are reprinted with permission from Clinical Dermatology, 2nd edition, by J. A. A. Hunter, J. A. Savin and M. V. Dahl, published 1995 by Blackwell Science, Oxford.

Figures 8.17 and 9.11 are reprinted with permission from *Textbook of Dermatology, 5th edition*, edited by R. H. Champion, J. L. Burton, F. J. G. Ebling, published 1992 by Blackwell Science, Oxford.

Figures 1.28, 1.59 and 4.36 are reprinted with permission from *Dermatology and the New Genetics*, by C. Moss and J. A. Savin, published 1995 by Blackwell Science, Oxford.

Figures 1.39 and 5.46 are reprinted with permission from *A Colour Atlas of Demonstrations in Surgical Pathology*, published 1986 by the Royal College of Surgeons/Wolfe Publishing Ltd., London.

We are also most grateful to Moira Gray for typing and retyping the manuscript, and to Jennifer Prast and the editorial staff at Mosby-Wolfe for their help and encouragement.

Introduction

There are two obvious ways of setting out an atlas on this topic. The first, and easiest, is to group pictures of the skin signs according to the underlying abnormality. One chapter would then deal with the changes seen in liver disease; another with those of renal disease; and so on. This approach would create a tidy book, but life is not like that.

In practice doctors are often faced with skin abnormalities which would ring no internal bells at all under the above arrangement and so they would have no idea which chapter to consult. With this in mind, we have preferred to base our chapters on the skin signs themselves, hoping that readers will be able to arrive quickly at a helpful page, where our text and pictures will guide them onward and perhaps inward.

Chapter 1 offers some possibilities to consider if the primary lesions can be identified. If not, then the most obvious feature may be the curious shape of the lesions (Chapter 2), an odd distribution (Chapters 3 and 4), a resemblance to one of the common dermatoses (Chapter 5), or an unusual colour (Chapter 6). The skin may have other characteristics, for example be too thin, too thick, too dry, too hairy etc. (Chapter 7), or react abnormally to its environment (Chapter 8). Finally, Chapter 9 is a reminder of skin problems which generate or are caused by abnormal skin sensation and Chapter 10 of lesions which crop up at various ages.

Of course a book of this size cannot cover all, or even most of the reputed 2000 skin disorders, each with its own range of presentations. We have therefore had to prune our original text and its illustrations considerably, and accept that others might have selected differently. Our final choices have been governed by two principles. First, conditions with general medical associations have been kept in at the expense of those which affect only the skin; and, second, common conditions have been given priority over rare ones.

Chapter 1

Lesions

The key to diagnosis lies in identifying primary lesions but this is not always easy. Often secondary changes such as scratch marks and infection dominate the picture. The secret is to find an early lesion, preferably an isolated one, away from the main eruption where primary and secondary lesions tend to make up a confusing jumble. Lighting should be uniform and bright and a magnifying lens helps to make subtle changes more obvious.

ERYTHEMA

Redness is one feature of a wide range of inflammatory skin disorders such as psoriasis. Less commonly it occurs alone.

Erythema per se may be localized as in the **palmar erythema** of pregnancy, liver disease (Fig. 1.1) or **graft versus host disease** (Fig. 1.2). **Facial flushing** is a feature of the **carcinoid syndrome** (Fig. 8.2). **Localized erythema** is also seen in some infections such as **erysipeloid** (Fig. 1.3) and **erysipelas** (Fig. 1.4), and in some **vascular naevi** (Fig. 1.5).

Erythema can also be **widespread** (erythroderma, Figs. 1.6 and 1.7). Causes include severe **atopic dermatitis and psoriasis, reactions to drugs** (Fig. 1.8), viral infections such as **measles** (Fig. 1.9) or **erythema infectiosum** (Fig. 1.10), with **bacterial toxaemia** (scarlet fever, the toxic shock syndrome) and as part of **connective tissue disorders** such as systemic lupus erythematosus or dermatomyositis (Fig. 1.11).

The features of **erythema multiforme** (Figs. 1.12 and 1.13), **erythema nodosum** (Fig. 1.14), and **erythema induratum** (Fig. 1.15), are important, distinctive and well-known — as are their internal causes. The annular erythemas are discussed on page 61.

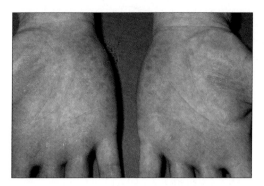

Fig. 1.1 Bilateral palmar erythema
Perhaps related to oestrogen, this occurs in several conditions including liver disease and pregnancy.

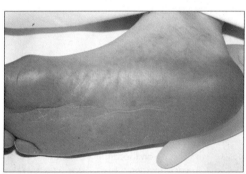

Fig. 1.2 Erythema of the palms and soles
This is an early cutaneous feature of graft versus host disease and in this case followed bone marrow transplantation.

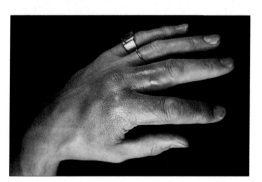

Fig. 1.3 Erysipeloid
The causative organism, erysipelothrix insidiosa, infects the hands of butchers and fishmongers. The organism is introduced through minor cuts.

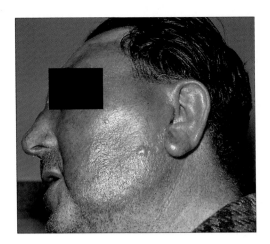

Fig. 1.4 Erysipelas

A small split under the lobe of one ear allowed this infection with β-haemolytic streptococci to gain entry. The condition tends to recur in the same place and is ushered in by fever and malaise before any eruption can be seen.

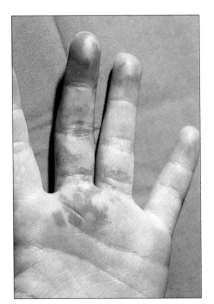

Fig. 1.5 Capillary haemangioma

A small and inconspicuous lesion, in this case unassociated with any underlying abnormality.

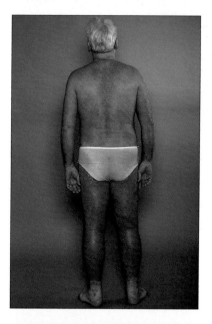

Fig. 1.6 Erythroderma
This patient's skin was red all over. Erythroderma can be due to extensive psoriasis, eczema, or drug eruptions, but in this case was due to pityriasis rubra pilaris. Protein loss, oedema, difficulty in controlling body temperature and occasionally high output cardiac failure may be seen.

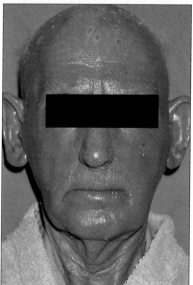

Fig. 1.7 Erythroderma
Unexplained erythroderma, as seen here, is sometimes due to an occult lymphoma.

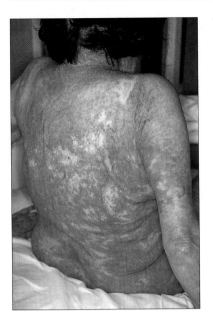

Fig. 1.8 Toxic erythema

This rather non-specific term covers a variety of patterns of erythema. In this case, the strange gyrate erythema, with some target-like lesions, seemed to be induced by penicillin.

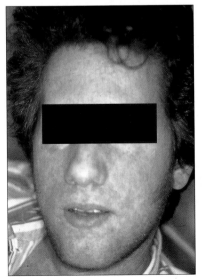

Fig. 1.9 Measles

Conjunctival infection appears early in the illness and the erythematous rash by the fourth day, fading and peeling over the next few days.

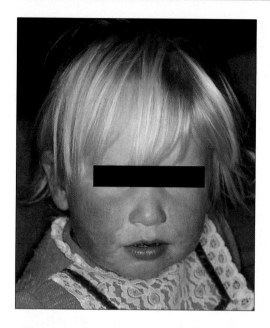

Fig. 1.10 Erythema infectiosum (fifth disease)
The 'slapped cheek' erythema of this human parvo-virus infection. Transient anaemia and arthritis may occur.

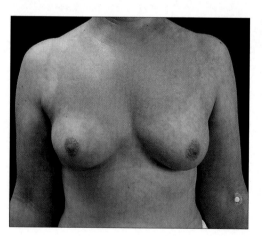

Fig. 1.11 Dermatomyositis
This patient presented with an unusually extensive erythema. Nail fold telangiectasia was also present.

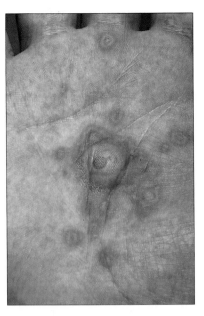

Fig. 1.12 Erythema multiforme
A typical example. Each target lesion has a peripheral red rim surrounding a pale centre. The bullseye is either erythematous or vesicular. This patient's attacks were triggered by recurrent herpes simplex infections. Systemic medication and other infections are also well known precipitants.

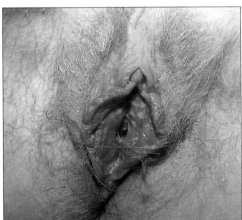

Fig. 1.13 Stevens–Johnson syndrome
Mucosal involvement is the most prominent feature (see also Fig. 1.82). Traditionally considered as a severe variant of erythema multiforme, some now believe it to be a separate entity caused by drugs.

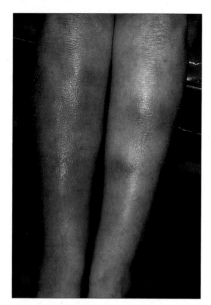

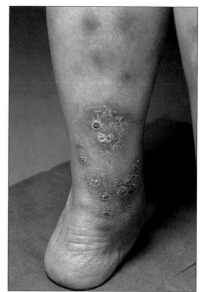

Fig. 1.14 Erythema nodosum
This is a reaction pattern, the internal causes of which are well known (the commonest being sarcoidosis, systemic medication, and infections, particularly with streptococci).

Fig. 1.15 Erythema induratum
Erythema induratum is usually seen in females with a chilblain tendency and puffy ankles. Underlying tuberculosis should be looked for but is not often found.

ERYTHEMATOSQUAMOUS ERUPTIONS

Here vascular dilatation is accompanied by scaling — both are signs of inflammation. Everyday causes include the common **inflammatory dermatoses** (e.g. eczema, psoriasis, pityriasis rosea and lichen planus), **infections** (fungi, candida and secondary syphilis) and **drug eruptions**.

A good clue to the diagnosis is often distribution. **Atopic eczema** will involve the flexor surfaces of the elbows and knees (Fig. 1.16), the wrists, face and the neck. **Seborrhoeic dermatitis** is common on the naso-labial folds and ears (Figs. 1.17 and 1.18). In contrast **psoriasis** favours the extensor aspects of major joints (Fig. 5.2) and the scalp (Fig. 4.18). In psoriasis the presence of nail changes (pitting, onycholysis and subungual hyperkeratosis) is often helpful (Fig. 4.54). The herald patch, collarettes of scales (Fig. 1.19), and the firtree distribution of

pityriasis rosea are characteristic. **Lichen planus** (Figs. 5.12–5.15) often involves the wrists and localizes to sites of trauma; this 'Koebnerization' is helpful also in psoriasis. Lichen planus also has a characteristic purplish colour.

Fungal infections are usually localized and unilateral (Figs. 1.20 and 1.21), in contrast to other conditions which tend to be symmetrical. **Secondary syphilis** (Fig. 1.22) is often widespread, and regularly involves the palms and soles. The most common type of **drug eruption** is a widespread erythema followed by scaling as it resolves (Fig.8.45). Similar eruptions can be caused by many **viral infections**.

The plaques of **discoid lupus erythematosus** are most common on the face (Fig. 1.23) and scalp. They are erythematous with scaling, follicular plugging (like a nutmeg grater) and sometimes scarring and atrophy. Systemic involvement is rare. Tender, pink scaly and atrophic plaques of the palms and soles (Fig. 1.24) are found in **subacute lupus erythematosus**, often with photosensitivity and a flitting arthropathy.

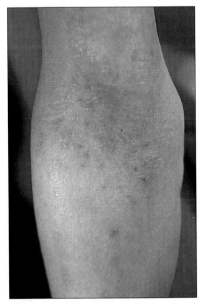

Fig. 1.16 Atopic eczema
The excoriations and lichenification (thickening of the skin and increased markings) are often most marked in the elbow flexures.

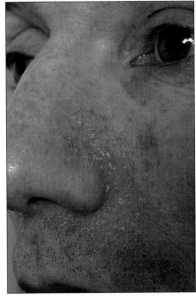

Fig. 1.17 Seborrhoeic dermatitis
Persistent redness and greasy scaling in this area may be an early sign of HIV infection.

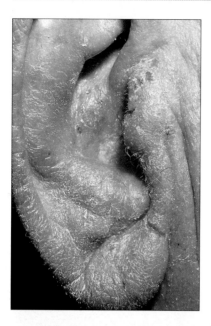

Fig. 1.18 Seborrhoeic dermatitis
Another favourite site for seborrhoeic dermatitis — sometimes combined with otitis externa.

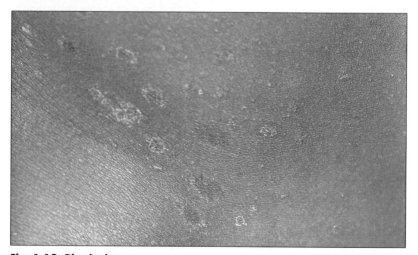

Fig. 1.19 Pityriasis rosea
The white scaly collarettes show up particularly well against the background racial pigmentation.

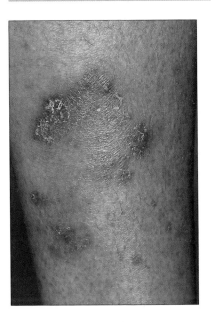

Fig. 1.20 Chronic fungal infection
These are characteristically annular, red
and scaly. Here the misguided use of
topical steroids has made the ring less
obvious. Follicular pustules are part of
'tinea incognito'.

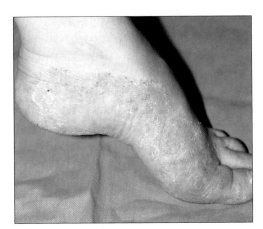

Fig. 1.21 Chronic fungal infection
The moccasin-type of chronic
tinea pedis is usually due to
trichophyton rubrum.

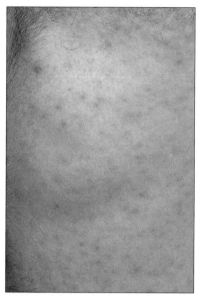

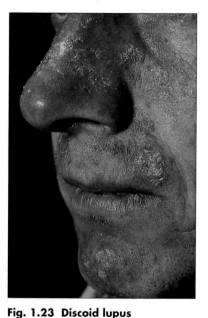

Fig. 1.22 Secondary syphilis
A symmetrical eruption, ham coloured but not itchy, with little scaling at this stage. Look for lesions on the palms and in the mouth.

Fig. 1.23 Discoid lupus erythematosus
Classical lesions on the face. The red scaly areas show marked follicular plugging.

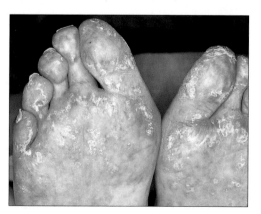

Fig. 1.24 Subacute lupus erythematosus
A similar combination of physical signs can be seen away from the face, here well demonstrated on the feet. The patient complained of intermittent pain and swelling of many large joints.

TELANGIECTASIA

Telangiectatic vessels are small and permanently dilated. They may be part of the weathering changes seen on elderly faces; less often they are clues to important internal disorders such as **mitral valve disease** (Fig. 1.25). In addition, telangiectasia is seen in many purely cutaneous disorders such as **rosacea** (Fig. 1.26), **discoid lupus erythematosus** (Fig.1.23) and **radiodermatitis** (Figs. 8.51 and 8.52). It is easy to see when skin atrophy is present, as in **poikiloderma** (Fig. 2.45) and after the excessive use of strong topical **corticosteroids** (Fig. 7.31). On the legs, arborizing telangiectasia may be a sign of **venous hypertension**.

Nail fold telangiectasia (Fig. 4.74) should never be ignored as it is a reliable pointer to an underlying **connective tissue disorder**, such as systemic lupus erythematosus, dermatomyositis, or systemic sclerosis. In the latter, telangiectatic mats are also commonly seen on the face (Fig. 1.27). These are similar to the lesions of **hereditary haemorrhagic telangiectasia** (Fig. 1.28) which must always be looked for in cases of severe recurrent nose or gut bleeding. **Angiokeratomas** (Fig. 1.29) are also an important clue to internal disease.

A typical **spider naevus** has a small, central, pulsatile 'body', surrounded by an area of erythema often showing telangiectatic 'legs' (Fig. 1.30) in which blood flows away from the centre. Many normal children and a few adults have one or two; more are seen during **pregnancy** and in **chronic liver disease** (Fig. 1.31), occasionally in a quasi-segmental distribution (**unilateral naevoid telangiectasia** (Fig. 3.19)).

Telangiectasia is also an early feature of one type of adult **cutaneous mastocytosis**; histamine release may then cause episodes of headache and flushing and there may also be systemic involvement (liver, spleen, bone and bone marrow). Telangiectasia is an early feature of **ataxia telangiectasia**, at first on the conjunctiva only but later also on the eyelids, cheeks and ears. The condition is rare but important as its other components include progressive ataxia and immunodeficiency.

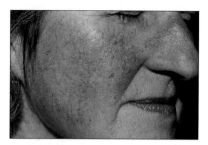

Fig. 1.25 Malar flush
Fixed, dilated telangiectatic vessels form
the basis of the characteristic malar flush
shown by this patient with mitral stenosis.
The telangiectasia which persists between
the flushing attacks of carcinoid can look
similar to this.

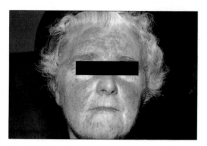

Fig. 1.26 Rosacea
A striking example. Typical features
include fixed erythema, telangiectasia,
papules and pustules. The condition was
worsened by the inappropriate use of
topical corticosteroids. This patient had an
associated blepharitis but never
developed keratoconjunctivitis.

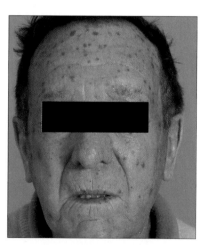

Fig. 1.27 Systemic sclerosis
This man with CREST variant showed
many small mat-like areas of
telangiectasia over his face and lips. His
nose was not beaked but the radial
furrowing around his mouth is typical.

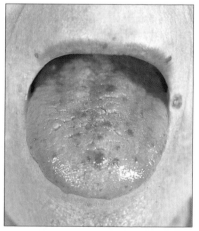

**Fig. 1.28 Hereditary
haemorrhagic telangiectasia**
This patient and many family members
had recurrent nose bleeds. Multiple small
telangiectatic lesions, most common on
the lips and tongue, are a good pointer to
the trait.

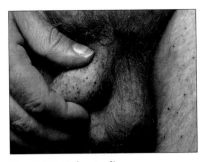

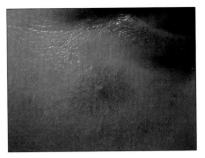

Fig. 1.29 Fabry's disease

Dark red telangiectatic papules appear characteristically on the scrotum but also may be more widespread. The condition is due to an inherited deficiency of the lysosomal enzyme α-galactosidase-A. Excruciating limb pain and vasomotor disturbances are other features of this condition which eventually leads to chronic renal failure.

Fig.1.30 Spider naevus

This patient had just one lesion. Pressure showed that it refilled from its slightly raised centre. The lesion cleared after light cautery to the central feeding arteriole. Multiple spider naevi are common in pregnancy and in chronic liver disease.

Fig. 1.31 Multiple spider naevi

These appeared in a patient with cirrhosis of the liver.

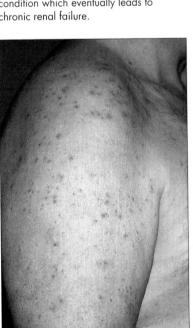

WHEALS

A typical wheal comes up after the intradermal injection of histamine; the release of histamine and other mediators of inflammation from dermal mast cells is the final common pathway in **urticaria** (Fig. 1.32). This release can be triggered in a variety of ways, many of which are non-allergic. Some are listed in Table 1. However, often it is not possible to identify the precise cause of an episode of urticaria.

Angioedema (Fig. 1.35) affects the subcutaneous tissues. It is not itchy and is less demarcated than the wheals of urticaria. The inherited varieties, due to abnormalities in C1 esterase inhibitor, carry the risk of fatal laryngeal oedema.

Table 1 The Main Types of Urticaria	
Physical	cold, solar, heat, cholinergic (Fig. 1.33), dermographism (Fig. 1.34), delayed pressure
Inherited	hereditary angioedema
Hypersensitivity	e.g. from shellfish or penicillin
Pharmacological	histamine releasers include aspirin and morphine derivatives
Contact	e.g. with animal saliva, some raw foods, caterpillars

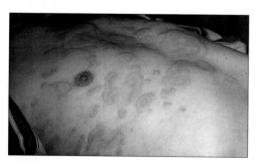

Fig. 1.32 Urticaria
Severe and acute whealing, triggered by a reaction to penicillin.
Reproduced with permission from Edwards, Bouchier, Haslett *et al* (eds), *Davidson's Principles and Practice of Medicine*, 17th edn., 1995, Churchill-Livingstone, Edinburgh.

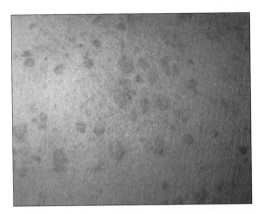

Fig.1.33 Cholinergic urticaria
Triggered by heat, exercise or anger, the small transient wheals are extremely itchy.

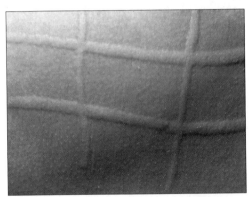

Fig.1.34 Immediate pressure urticaria (dermographism)
Transient whealing in response to minor pressure affects a small proportion of the population. It may be a lifelong tendency, giving no symptoms, or acquired, in which case itching from minor skin trauma can be distressing.

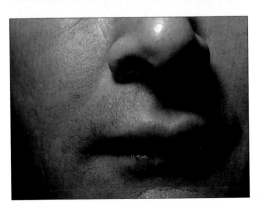

Fig.1.35 Angioedema
The dangerous but rare inherited type is an autosomal dominant trait and due to a functional deficiency of C1 esterase inhibitor. Laryngeal obstruction is a real risk. This patient had the non-inherited type which, unlike the inherited type, occurs in association with straight- forward itchy wheals or urticaria elsewhere on the skin.

PURPURA AND VASCULITIS

Purpura, the result of leakage of red blood cells into the skin (Fig. 1.36), are purple to brown macules or papules, often most prominent on the lower legs, which fail to blanch in response to pressure. The smallest are **petechiae** and the largest **ecchymoses**. Coagulation disorders give rise to ecchymoses (Figs. 1.37 and 1.38) and external bleeding, whereas platelet and vessel wall defects cause petechiae.

Purpura is either **thrombocytopenic** or **non-thrombocytopenic**. The former may be idiopathic, a feature of connective tissue disorders (especially lupus erythematosus), due to bone marrow damage (e.g. cytotoxic drugs, leukaemia), or to drugs (e.g. quinine, aspirin, thiazides, sulphonamides).

Damage to vessels is responsible for non-thrombocytopenic purpura. It may be mechanical as in talon noir (Fig. 1.39). Poor vascular support by the surrounding dermis underlies the purpura seen after minor trauma to elderly skin (Fig. 7.27); as a side effect of **potent topical corticosteroids**; in **systemic amyloidosis** (Figs. 7.48 and 7.49) and in **scurvy**. Purpura may accompany any inflammation of the lower legs.

Vessels can also be damaged by infections (e.g. **meningococcal septicaemia** (Fig. 1.40) and some **drug reactions** (e.g. thiazides, carbromal and quinine).

Vasculitis — inflammation of blood vessels — has a host of manifestations depending on the size, type and location of the vessels affected. It is not a diagnosis in itself, but part of a range of pathological processes. Many tissues can be affected, but the skin, because of its profuse vascular supply and ready visiblilty, is often where it is first recognized, usually on the lower legs. Unfortunately no clinical pattern is specific to any underlying cause.

In acute vasculitis of small vessels (e.g. **Henoch–Schönlein purpura** (Fig. 1.41)), the purpura are often slightly raised and indurated — so called 'painful palpable purpura' (Fig. 1.42). Often this is an immunological reaction to an infection, (e.g. hepatitis B, streptococci, or CMV), a drug (e.g. aspirin or penicillin) or a systemic disease (e.g. SLE, rheumatoid arthritis or inflammatory bowel disease). If larger vessels are involved, tender nodules develop, as in **polyarteritis nodosa**.

Urticarial vasculitis differs from common urticaria as individual lesions last longer than 24 hours and leave bruises behind. Although this is usually idiopathic, SLE should always be considered.

Other vasculitic reaction patterns include **erythema nodosum** (Fig. 1.14) and **erythema induratum** (Fig. 1.15). The causes of erythema nodosum include streptococcal infections, medications such as sulphonamides, inflammatory bowel disease, tuberculosis and sarcoidosis.

Necrosis may be a prominent feature, the first manifestation being haemorrhagic blisters which ulcerate, often leaving a hard black eschar (Fig.1.41).

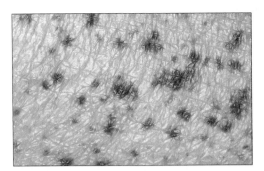

Fig. 1.36 Purpuric eruption

This florid purpuric eruption seemed to be drug-induced, perhaps being a response to a dextran infusion.

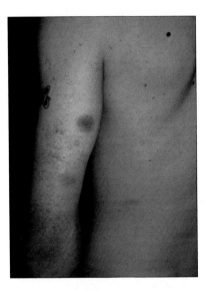

Fig. 1.37 Ecchymoses

Spontaneous ecchymoses were the presenting feature of thrombocytopenia here.

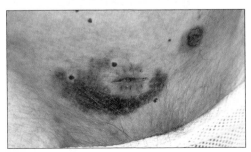

Fig. 1.38 Ecchymoses

Ecchymoses round a biopsy site, in a patient who had taken aspirin regularly for cardiac reasons. The bruising is least obvious by the wound itself where the tissues were held tightly together by suturing.

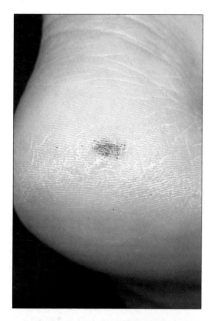

Fig. 1.39 Talon noir
This surgeon plays squash but was
relieved to hear that this speckled
pigmentation was purpuric and not due to
melanin. Paring removed his lesion.

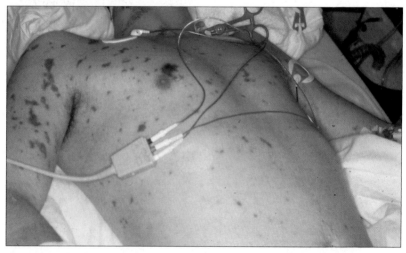

Fig. 1.40 Meningococcal septicaemia
Erythematous, rapidly becoming purpuric, the eruption may help in making an early
diagnosis in this potentially lethal condition.

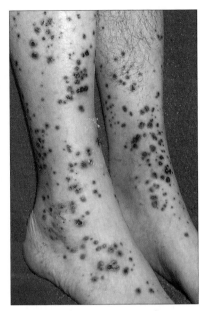

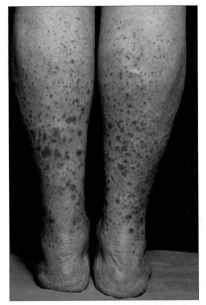

Fig. 1.41 Cutaneous vasculitis
Painful purpura, becoming necrotic. Look
for renal, gut and joint involvement
(Henoch Schönlein type).

Fig. 1.42 Cutaneous vasculitis
Palpable purpura — in this patient due to
a drug.

MACULES AND PAPULES

A **macule** is a small (less than 0.5 cm across), flat area of altered colour or texture.
A **papule** is a small (less than 0.5 cm across), solid elevation of the skin.

The terms are useful for describing skin lesions, but not particularly useful
diagnostically as most eruptions consist of macules (e.g. café au lait macules (Fig.
6.2)), or papules (e.g. **molluscum contagiosum** (Fig. 1.43)), **Campbell de Morgan
spots** (Fig. 1.44) and **diffuse granuloma annulare** (Fig. 1.45), or a mixture of the
two. But occasionally the appearance of some papules points to important
underlying disorders (e.g. **Gottron's papules** (Figs. 2.41 and 5.18), **lichen
myxoedematosus** (Fig. 1.46) and **xanthomata** (Figs. 6.31 and 6.32)).

Examples can be found on almost every page of this book.

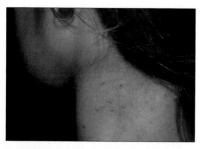

Fig. 1.43 Molluscum contagiosum
The papules of molluscum contagiosum here are scattered over the back of the neck. Some show the typical central keratotic plug. There is a patchy background erythema. Intractible lesions occur with atopic eczema and with AIDS.

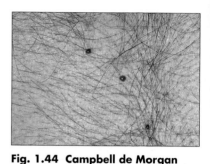

Fig. 1.44 Campbell de Morgan spots
A scattering of these small benign haemangiomas is not uncommon in the middle-aged and elderly but does not imply any underlying disease.

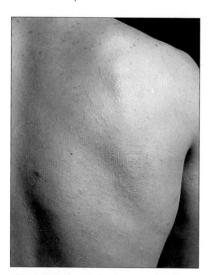

Fig. 1.45 Granuloma annulare
This diffuse type, with numerous tiny papules, is more likely to be associated with diabetes than the ordinary annular type seen on the fingers of children.

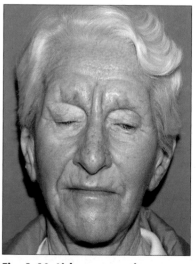

Fig. 1.46 Lichen myxoedematosus (scleromyxoedema)
Deposits of mucin are responsible for the papules seen on the upper part of the forehead and for the thickening above the eyebrows. A monoclonal paraproteinaemia is invariably present.

NODULES

A **nodule** is a solid mass in the skin, usually greater than 0.5 cm in diameter. Good examples include the nodules of **rheumatoid arthritis** (Fig. 1.47), of **lepromatous leprosy** (Fig. 1.48), of some cutaneous **tumours** (e.g. the nodular type of melanoma (Fig.1.69)), secondary deposits (Figs. 1.79 and 1.80), lymphomas (Fig. 1.49), nodular prurigo and even dermatofibroma (Fig. 1.50).

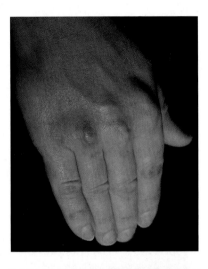

Fig. 1.47 Rheumatoid nodule
Small lesion present on the knuckle of a patient with early rheumatoid arthritis.

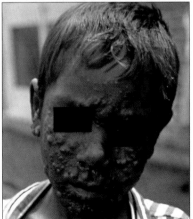

Fig. 1.48 Lepromatous leprosy
Numerous facial nodules can be seen, typical of this diagnosis.

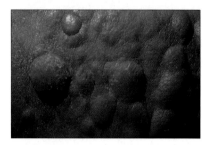

Fig. 1.49 Cutaneous B cell lymphoma
Cutaneous nodules were the presenting feature of this aggressive and rapidly fatal lymphoma.

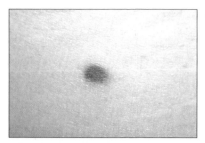

Fig. 1.50 Dermatofibroma
Common and benign, these lesions are indurated and attached to the epidermis — hence the hint of dimpling which becomes more obvious if the surrounding skin is pinched. The pigment is a mixture of melanin and haemosiderin.

GRANULOMAS

This is a pathological term, but one which has also a clinical meaning. Granulomas form when cell-mediated immunity fails to eliminate antigen. They arise, for instance, when organisms cannot be destroyed, as in **tuberculosis** (Fig. 1.51), **leishmaniasis** (Fig. 1.52), **leprosy** (Fig. 1.53), and when a foreign substance cannot be eliminated (e.g. **tattoo granulomas** (Fig. 6.34)). In many cases the cause has yet to be determined, as in **rosacea**, **granuloma annulare** and **sarcoidosis** (Fig. 1.54).

The clinical features are those of a slowly spreading chronic inflammation with indurated plaques, papules and even pustules. A typical brownish colour is best seen using diascopy (i.e. viewing the lesion which is being pressed on by a glass slide).

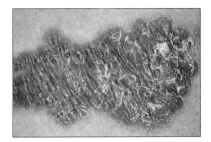

Fig. 1.51 Lupus vulgaris
This chronic plaque, with scaling and atrophic wrinkling, has a characteristic reddish-brown colour, and diascopy showed apple jelly colour. The lesion had been present for many years but cleared well with standard anti-tuberculosis therapy.

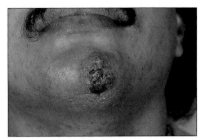

Fig. 1.52 Leishmaniasis
This patient from the Middle East had been bitten by a sandfly three months previously. A biopsy allowed the parasite to be demonstrated with Giemsa's stain. The lesion cleared slowly over six months leaving some scarring.

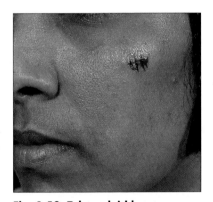

Fig. 1.53 Tuberculoid leprosy
A characteristic area of hypopigmentation and sensory impairment. Biopsy and look for thickening of local nerves.

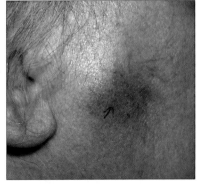

Fig. 1.54 Sarcoidosis
Typical plum-coloured indurated plaque of sarcoidosis.

TUMOURS

Benign skin tumours are common and include viral (Figs. 5.39–5.41) and seborrhoeic warts (Figs. 5.45 and 5.46), keratoacanthomas (Fig. 1.55), dermatofibromas (Fig. 1.50), lipomas (Fig. 1.56), neurofibromas and melanocytic naevi (Figs. 1.57 and 1.58). They seldom indicate internal disease, exceptions being **multiple neurofibromas** (Figs. 3.23, 6.2 and 6.3) and the sudden appearance of numerous itchy, seborrhoeic warts which may suggest internal malignancy (the sign of Leser–Trélat). Skin tags (acrochordons) (Fig.5.52) are especially common in the obese and in **tuberous sclerosis**, acanthosis nigricans, acromegaly and diabetes. Angiofibromas, clustered around the nose (Fig. 1.59) and on the cheeks may signal tuberous sclerosis (Fig. 1.60). Congenital sweat and sebaceous gland tumours on the scalp (Fig. 1.61) are most often benign but basal cell carcinomas develop in about 25% in later life. Numerous and highly **resistant viral warts** may be seen in immunodeficient patients such as after a renal transplant, or with sarcoidosis (Fig. 5.41), a lymphoma, or AIDS.

The three commonest **malignant tumours** are **basal** (Figs. 1.62–1.64) and **squamous cell carcinomas** (Figs. 1.65–1.67 and 4.52) and **malignant melanomas** (Figs. 1.68 and 1.69). The first two relate to chronic sun damage and ageing. The exception is the melanoma which may be triggered by periods of intense sun exposure. In young patients, a predisposing cause for malignant tumours, such as albinism (Fig. 4.16), xeroderma pigmentosum (Figs. 8.22 and 8.23) or Gorlin's syndrome (Fig. 1.70), should be considered.

Many **vascular tumours**, such as Campbell de Morgan spots (Fig. 1.44) and pyogenic granulomas (Fig. 1.71), are benign. However, **Kaposi's sarcoma** (Fig. 1.72), a malignant tumour of proliferating capillaries and lymphatics, now thought to be due to Herpes virus type 8, may be associated with AIDS. Atypical lesions often resemble bruises (Fig. 1.73).

Lymphomas and leukaemias may affect the skin (Fig. 1.74), forming patches, plaques, nodules and then ulcers. The skin is involved early in **mycosis fungoides** (Fig. 1.75) which may be limited to it for many years. Persistent red scaly plaques on the breast and perianal area should alert physicians to examine for an underlying carcinoma which has involved the skin (Figs. 1.76–1.78). The skin is a relatively uncommon and late site for **secondary tumours** and only a small minority of those with internal malignancy develop cutaneous metastases. Two favourite sites are the umbilicus (Fig. 1.79) and the scalp (Fig. 1.80). Solitary nodules are the most common manifestation but firm areas of erythema, telangiectatic plaques and papules also occur. Flat telangiectatic areas of hair loss may be due to secondary deposits from carcinoma of the breast and, overall, the breast is the most common primary site, followed by the lung, GI tract, uterus, prostate and kidney.

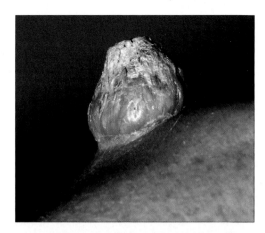

**Fig. 1.55
Keratoacanthoma**
A rapidly growing tumour with a characteristic morphology. These tumours always look alike with a central keratin plug within a fleshy surround. These features separate them from the squamous cell carcinomas which they resemble histologically.

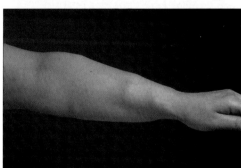

Fig. 1.56 Lipoma
Multiple subcutaneous lesions can easily be seen here.

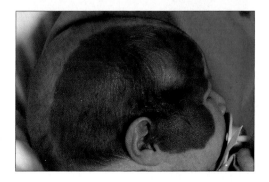

Fig. 1.57 Congenital melanocytic naevus
The twin risks here are an associated involvement of the meninges and transition into a malignant melanoma.

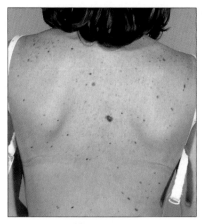

Fig. 1.58 Melanocytic naevi
A deliberately distant view to show
numbers but not detail — the more naevi,
the greater the risk of a melanoma
developing. The largest lesion in the
centre of the back is an invasive, nodular
melanoma (see Fig. 1.69).

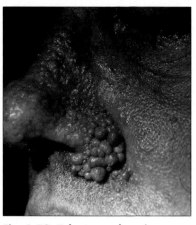

Fig. 1.59 Tuberous sclerosis
Gross angiofibromas ('adenoma
sebaceum') clustering around the nose in
a patient with tuberous sclerosis.

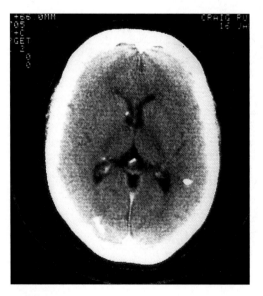

Fig. 1.60 Cortical tubers
Cortical tubers (white) seen on
a CT scan of a patient with
tuberous sclerosis.

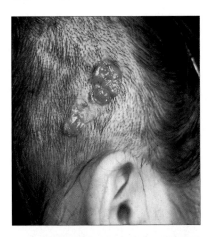

Fig. 1.61 Naevus sebaceus and syringocystadenoma papilliferum

A solitary yellow hairless area, the naevus sebaceus, had been present on the scalp since birth. This exuberant but benign papillomatous tumour, an apocrine hamartoma, developed on top of it after many years. Multiple sebaceous naevi may be one component of the epidermal naevus syndrome which includes abnormalities of the CNS, eyes and skeleton (see Fig. 2.36).

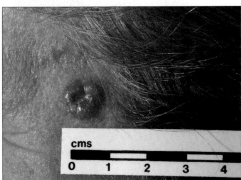

Fig. 1.62 Basal cell carcinoma

This small lesion has not yet ulcerated; its sunken centre emphasizes the classical shiny, translucent quality of the rest of the lesion.

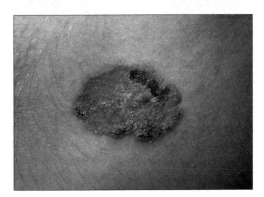

Fig. 1.63 Superficial basal cell carcinoma

The thin shiny translucent, beaded rim around this lesion becomes even more obvious when the skin is stretched. Nevertheless, the diagnosis of superficial basal cell carcinoma is often missed.

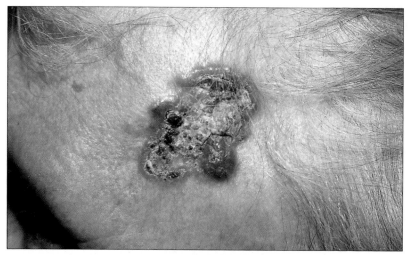

Fig. 1.64 Basal cell carcinoma
The rolled edge of this basal cell carcinoma is obvious at the upper pole of the lesion; but the family doctor was distracted by the heavy pigmentation and was worried about the possibility of a melanoma.

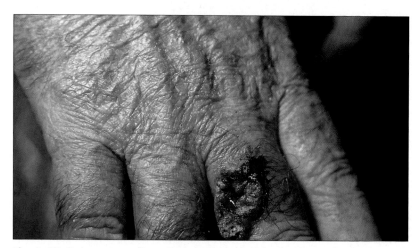

Fig. 1.65 Squamous cell carcinoma The back of this hand is wrinkled and atrophic after many years of sun exposure which must also have played a part in causing this rapidly growing tumour.

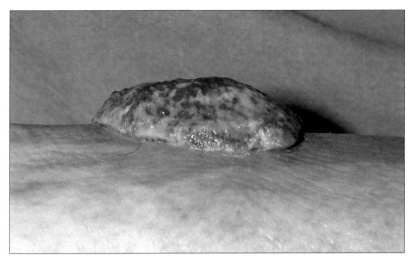

Fig. 1.66 Squamous cell carcinoma This rapidly growing, friable, raised tumour was confirmed by biopsy as a squamous cell carcinoma.

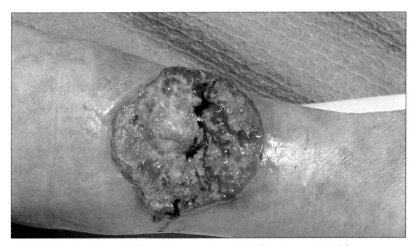

Fig. 1.67 Squamous cell carcinoma This massive lesion was treated for many months as a stasis ulcer. However, it was raised rather than depressed, and its histology was that of an ulcerated squamous cell carcinoma.

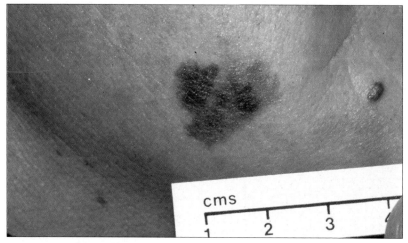

Fig. 1.68 Lentigo maligna
The characteristic mixture of different shades of pigmentation is well shown in this lesion which carries a significant risk of changing into an invasive malignant melanoma.

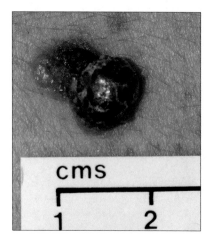

Fig. 1.69 Nodular malignant melanoma
All of the ABCDE criteria of malignant melanoma are satisfied (**A**symmetry, **B**order irregularity, **C**olour variability, **D**iameter greater than 0.5cm, **E**levation irregularity).Same patient as in Fig. 1.58.

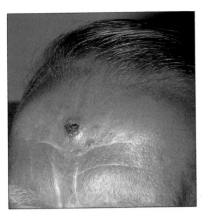

Fig. 1.70 Gorlin's syndrome

The reflection on this patient's forehead emphasizes the frontal bossing which is characteristic of Gorlin's syndrome (basal cell naevus syndrome). He has one current basal cell carcinoma and shows the scars where others have been removed in the past. The condition should be suspected if a young person develops one or more basal cell carcinomas. It is inherited as an autosomal dominant trait, the other features of which include dental cysts and skeletal abnormalities such as bifid ribs.

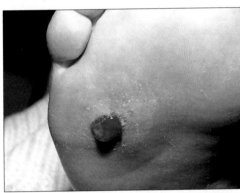

Fig. 1.71 Pyogenic granuloma

These vascular tumours bleed easily even if they are not on the sole. Always check the histology to exclude an amelanotic melanoma.

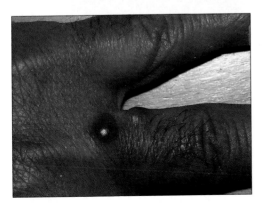

Fig. 1.72 Kaposi's sarcoma

These dusky nodules on the hand of a middle aged, middle European male were of the 'classical' type, unassociated with an HIV infection.

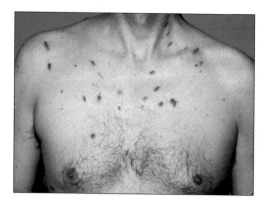

Fig. 1.73 Kaposi's sarcoma
These bruise-like lesions all came up within a few weeks in a homosexual patient with AIDS.

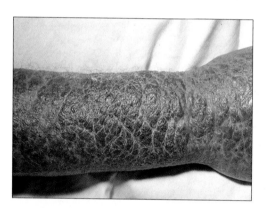

Fig. 1.74 Leukaemic infiltration
Biopsy confirmed that these extensive purple plaques in a patient with established chronic lymphatic leukaemia were due to leukaemic infiltration.

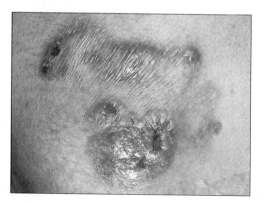

Fig. 1.75 Cutaneous T cell lymphoma (mycosis fungoides)
This infiltrated plaque, with a typical arciform outline, arose on a persistent area of erythema, scaling and atrophy (the pre-mycotic eruption) which can still be seen in the background.

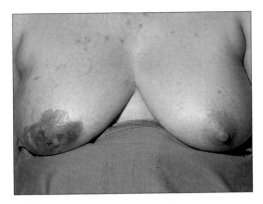

Fig. 1.76 Paget's disease
The architecture of the right nipple has been destroyed by a slowly expanding reddish marginated plaque. An underlying intraductal carcinoma of the breast should be looked for. The left nipple is unaffected.

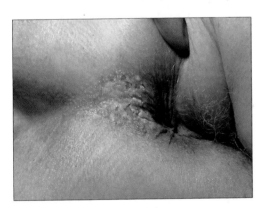

Fig. 1.77 Extramammary Paget's disease
Biopsy showed that this macerated perianal plaque was due to extra-mammary Paget's disease. An underlying carcinoma of the rectum was found. See also Fig. 4.80.

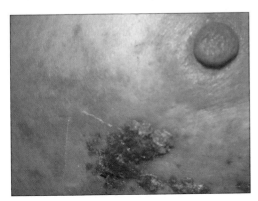

Fig. 1.78 Carcinoma of the breast
The obvious raised tumour is a breast cancer invading the overlying skin. Around it can be seen pink telangiectatic areas, also due to direct invasion (carcinoma telangiectoides).

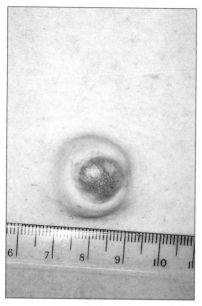

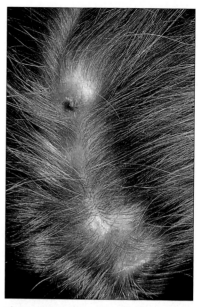

Fig. 1.79 Umbilical secondary (Sister Joseph's nodule)
May appear before other manifestations of an intra-abdominal carcinoma, usually a gastric one.

Fig. 1.80 Scalp secondaries
Hard lumps in the elderly scalp may be blood-borne metastases.

ULCERS AND EROSIONS

An **ulcer** is an area from which the whole epidermis and at least part of the dermis has been lost. Ulcers may be deep and even extend through to the subcutaneous fat; they heal with scarring. **Erosions** are denuded areas with a complete or partial loss of the epidermis alone; they heal without scarring. Superficial discrete and glistening erosions are seen in various types of **pemphigus** and **pemphigoid** (Figs. 1.81 and 1.106) and in the Stevens–Johnson syndrome, a severe variant of **erythema multiforme** (Fig. 1.82).

Vascular disease underlies most ulcers. **Venous hypertension** accounts for some 85% of leg ulcers, most commonly near the medial malleolus (Fig. 1.83). Other signs include a red or bluish discolouration, loss of hair, induration, haemosiderin pigmentation and atrophie blanche (areas of ivory white scarring with dilated capillaries (Fig. 1.84)).

Atherosclerotic ulcers (Fig. 1.85), most common on the toes, dorsum of the foot, heel, calf and shin, are sharply defined, may be deep and are accompanied by absent pulses, intermittent claudication and nocturnal cramps. They are a feature of the rare premature ageing condition, **Werner's syndrome** (Fig. 1.86). Vasculitic ulcers, in **rheumatoid arthritis** (Fig. 1.87) and other connective tissue disorders, start as painful palpable purpuric lesions, which later turn into necrotic ulcers. **Sickle cell anaemia** and **cryoglobulinaemia** are other causes of recalcitrant leg ulcers.

Ulceration of the sole (Fig. 9.11), especially if accompanied by paraesthesia or anaesthesia, is likely to be due to the neuropathy of diabetes or leprosy and less often to syphilis or syringomyelia.

Ulcers may be due to **infection**. Good examples are the early and late lesions of syphilis (Figs. 1.88 and 1.89) but other bacteria may be equally responsible (Fig. 1.90). Persistent leg ulcers are common in the tropics. '**Tropical ulcer**' (an infection with Fusobacterium species and spirochaetes or anaerobes, tuberculosis and deep fungal infections) should be considered.

A hyperplastic granulating base or edge should raise the suspicion of **malignancy**. In this context, squamous cell carcinoma (Fig. 1.67) is a more common cause than basal cell carcinoma (Figs. 1.91 and 1.92), malignant melanoma (Fig. 1.69 and 1.58) or lymphoma.

An **artefact** (Fig. 1.93) should be suspected in persistent bizarre ulceration in a young and miserable woman, even though her over-protective parent may have been hoodwinked ('folie a deux'). But not all curiosities, including chrome ulceration (Fig. 1.94) are artefactual.

In **pyoderma gangrenosum** (Figs. 1.120–1.122), pustules turn into large and rapidly spreading ulcers which are often circular or polycyclic and have a blue, undermined or pustular margin. This condition may be seen with rheumatoid arthritis, ulcerative colitis and blood dyscrasias.

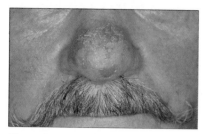

Fig. 1.81 Pemphigus erythematosus

The superficial blisters of this condition have a thin roof which ruptures rapidly leaving shallow erosions, as seen here on the nose.

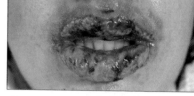

Fig. 1.82 Stevens–Johnson syndrome

Haemorrhagic crusting and erosions of the lips are an important part of this syndrome (see also Fig. 4.43).

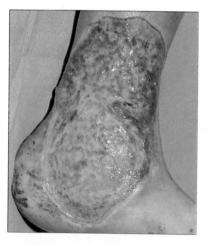

Fig. 1.83 Venous ulceration

The punched out edge shows that this venous ulcer is not healing. The greenish colour of the sloughy base suggests a super-added pseudomonas infection.

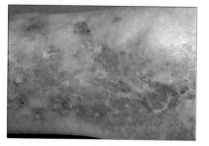

Fig. 1.84 Atrophie blanche

The reticulate arrangement of ivory-white areas is well seen. Minor trauma leads to persistent and painful ulceration.

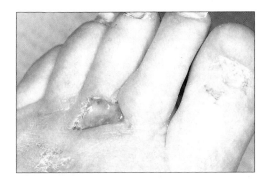

Fig. 1.85 An arterial ulcer
A cold foot, with absent pulses and ulceration at the base of the toes rather than in the classical venous areas.

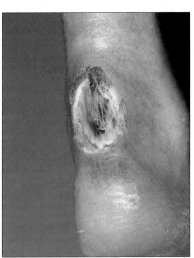

Fig. 1.86 Werner's syndrome
Atherosclerotic leg ulcers, here shown reaching down to the Achilles tendon, are a common part of this rare premature ageing syndrome. Early greying of the hair, sclerodactyly, diabetes, cataracts and a tendency to internal malignancy are also seen.

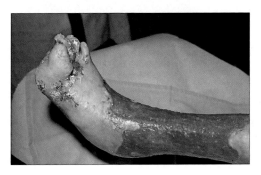

Fig. 1.87 Rheumatoid arthritis
Extensive ulcers form easily around the ankle and heal poorly. Immobility and an underlying vasculitis both contribute to this.

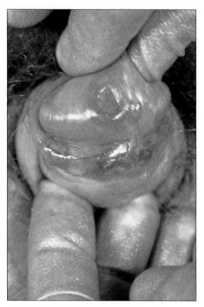

Fig. 1.88 Primary chancre
Ulcerated chancres can be seen here, on the glans and on the coronal sulcus.

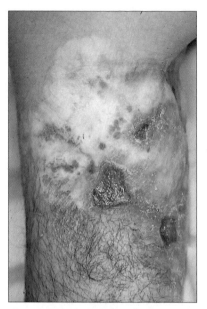

Fig. 1.89 Gummata
The punched out ulcers were due to late syphilis and occurred in an area of variably pigmented atrophic scarring.

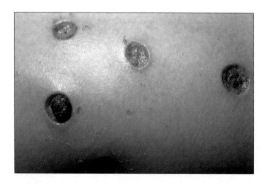

Fig. 1.90 Ecthyma
A scattering of punched out ulcers, some with a central black eschar, followed a streptococcal infection of neglected insect bites.

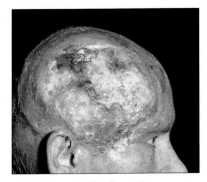

Fig. 1.91 Basal cell carcinoma
A neglected basal cell carcinoma which took five years to penetrate down to the meninges.

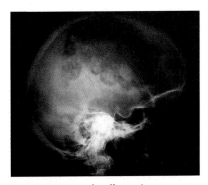

Fig. 1.92 Basal cell carcinoma
The skull X-ray of the same patient showing precisely where the tumour had destroyed bone.

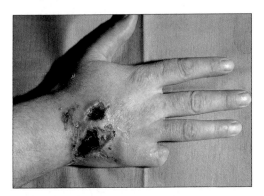

Fig. 1.93 Artefactual ulcers
These were caused by self-applications of a corrosive fluid; the motive remained obscure.

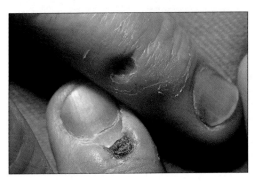

Fig. 1.94 Chrome ulcers
This patient was an electroplater, in contact with corrosive chrome salts which were responsible for the way minor cuts on his fingers changed into persistent ulcers. The proximal nail fold is a typical site; perforation of the nasal septum may also occur.

NECROSIS

Large areas of necrosis are a sinister, but rare sign. **Necrotizing fasciitis** (Fig. 1.95) is caused by a mixture of pathogens, usually including streptococci and anaerobes. Lesions most commonly on the head and neck, start as hot, tender erythematous or dusky swellings. Only when blistering and a rapidly extending necrosis occur is the urgency of the situation appreciated. Immediate and extensive surgical debridement is required, with intravenous benzylpenicillin and metronidazole. **Progressive synergistic gangrene** around a recent surgical wound is a form of necrotizing fasciitis which requires the same prompt treatment. The herpes virus, varicella zoster, can also cause necrosis (Fig. 1.96).

   Necrolytic migratory erythema (Fig. 2.3) is a rare but distinctive cutaneous reaction which accompanies an underlying **glucagonoma**. Waves of shifting erythema, most often on the lower trunk, show superficial necrosis, crusting and desquamation and leave pigmentation in their wake.

   Cutaneous necrosis (Fig. 1.97) is a rare side effect of **coumarin anticoagulants** especially warfarin. Fatty areas (e.g. the breasts, buttocks, thighs, abdomen) are most often affected, usually within two weeks of starting treatment. An inherited protein C deficiency is sometimes found.

   Gangrene is most common on the limbs of the elderly. **Thrombosis or embolism**, secondary to atherosclerosis, causes infarction of the skin. Digital gangrene may complicate arterial disease in **diabetes** (Fig. 1.99). **Frostbite** (Fig. 1.98) is another cause of gangrene. The digits are most commonly affected and old age, peripheral vascular disease, **cryoglobulinaemia** (Figs. 8.41 and 8.42) and smoking are predisposing factors.

   Necrosis may also occur in **tumours** (Fig. 1.100) when their growth outstrips their blood supply.

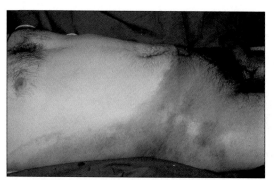

Fig. 1.95 Necrotizing fasciitis
Within 24 hours a small but tender area of perineal inflammation spread to this extent. The patient survived but only after emergency radical excisional surgery.

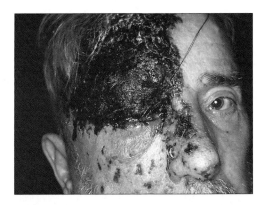

Fig. 1.96 Ophthalmic zoster
Unusually haemorrhagic and necrotic, with some spread outside the main segment — investigations are needed to exclude underlying immunodeficiency, as in AIDS, leukaemia or a lymphoma.

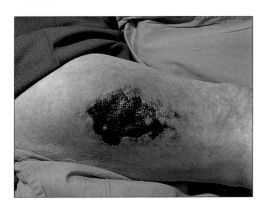

Fig. 1.97 Cutaneous necrosis
Here seen in a patient on warfarin.

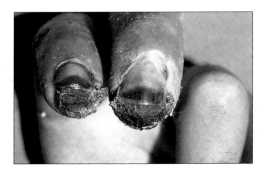

Fig. 1.98 Gangrene of the finger tips
In this case due to frostbite.

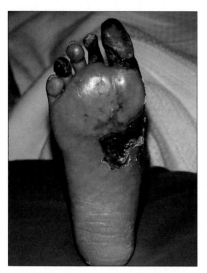

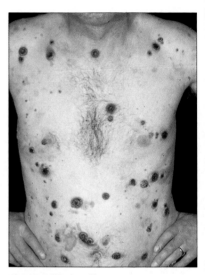

Fig. 1.99 Gangrene of the foot
This extensive gangrene of the foot
occurred in a patient with diabetes mellitus.

**Fig. 1.100 T cell cutaneous
lymphoma**
The tumour stage of a T cell cutaneous
lymphoma. Many of the tumours have
spontaneously become necrotic.

BLISTERS

The skin is made up of several layers and when these separate the level of the
split can often be deduced clinically. Blisters arising beneath the epidermis, for
example, may contain blood and have roofs thick enough to prevent easy rupture.
Such sub-epidermal blisters often have erythema around them and heal with
scarring and sometimes with **milia** formation (Fig. 1.129).

The various types of **epidermolysis bullosa** illustrate these principles well. All
are inherited disorders of skin cohesion. They are divided into **simplex, dystrophic**
and **junctional** types (Figs. 1.101, 1.102 and 8.26) in which blisters occur
respectively in the epidermis (keratin abnormalities), dermis (anchoring fibril
abnormalities) and at the dermo-epidermal junction (anchoring filament
abnormalities).

Other blisters with an intra-epidermal origin include those of **pemphigus vulgaris** (Fig. 1.103) and **pemphigus erythematosus** (Figs. 1.104 and 1.105), both acquired autoimmune disorders. Their blisters rupture so easily that often only erosions are seen. In contrast, **pemphigoid**, also an autoimmune disorder, has thick roofed sub-epidermal blisters, often on an erythematous base (Fig. 1.106). The blisters of **dermatitis herpetiformis**, though sub-epidermal, are so itchy that they are quickly broken by scratching. They come up in groups, mainly on the extensor surfaces of the elbows and knees and on the shoulders, buttocks and scalp (Figs. 1.107 and 1.108), and are associated with gluten hypersensitivity.

Blistering is also important in **inflammatory disorders** such as eczema (Fig. 1.109), fungal infections (Figs. 1.20 and 1.21), lichen planus (Figs. 5.12–5.15), bullous impetigo and the staphylococcal scalded skin syndrome (Figs. 1.110 and 8.27). Blisters are also obvious in shingles (Fig. 1.111), herpes simplex infections (Figs. 1.112 and 1.113), hand foot and mouth disease (Fig. 1.114), and as a response to insect bites (Fig. 1.115) and jellyfish stings. Sometimes blistering is drug-provoked; if it occurs repeatedly at the same site, a fixed drug eruption (Fig. 1.116) should be suspected. In **porphyria cutanea tarda**, the skin on exposed parts becomes fragile and blisters easily (Figs. 8.18 and 8.19).

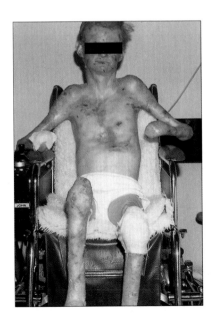

Fig. 1.101 Epidermolysis bullosa; autosomal recessive dystrophic type
The minor trauma of everyday life is enough to produce massive blisters which heal with scarring. This resulted in loss of the digits of the hands and feet. The teeth may be malformed. Blistering and subsequent scarring of the oral and upper oesophageal mucosa often occur. Life becomes a mere existence for those severely affected.

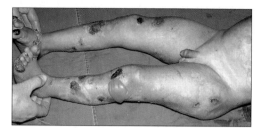

Fig. 1.102 Epidermolysis bullosa; junctional type
Minor trauma has again produced large blisters and erosions which heal slowly or not at all. The condition is often fatal.

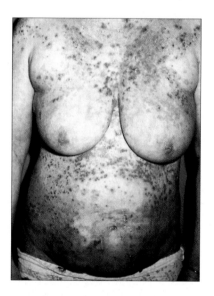

Fig. 1.103 Pemphigus vulgaris
An extensive eruption with numerous scattered crusted erosions and a few flaccid blisters on a background of erythema. Histology and immunofluorescence confirmed the diagnosis.

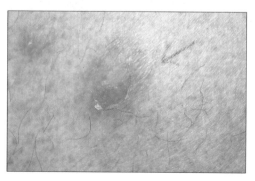

Fig. 1.104 Pemphigus erythematosus
The blisters of pemphigus erythematosus arise even more superficially within the epidermis than those of pemphigus vulgaris. They break early leaving crusted erosions. These are typical and were confirmed by biopsy.

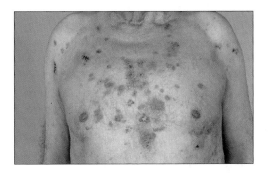

Fig. 1.105 Pemphigus erythematosus
This patient shows the typical erythematous erosions of pemphigus erythematosus on his upper chest. Blisters are hard to see.

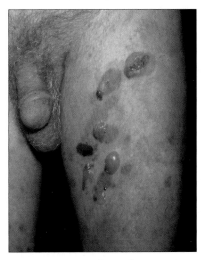

Fig. 1.106 Pemphigoid
These are subepidermal blisters. Often, as here, they become large and tense without breaking. Some arise on urticarial plaques. The condition, which usually affects the elderly, may remit after months or years; until then immunosuppressive therapy is needed. An association with internal malignancy is still debated.

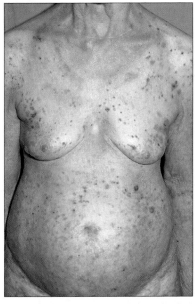

Fig. 1.107 Dermatitis herpetiformis
Dapsone rapidly suppressed this itchy vesicular eruption and could be tapered off 6 months after the patient had gone on a gluten-free diet. This will have to be continued for life to control skin symptoms and to reduce the risk of developing a small bowel lymphoma.

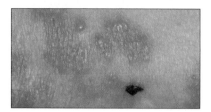

Fig 1.108 Dermatitis herpetiformis
The tiny subepidermal blisters are arranged in groups on a red background. Favourite sites include the points of the elbows and knees, and the shoulder blades.

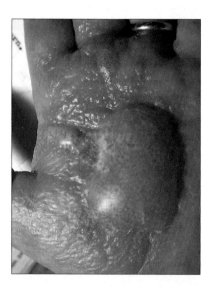

Fig. 1.109 Acute contact dermatitis
Antihistamines are good sensitizers when used topically. This patient developed an acute contact dermatitis, of the palm and elsewhere, after applying an antihistamine cream to an area of sunburn. The artificiality of the distinction between vesicles and bullae is well illustrated here; the main blister is multiloculated and intact vesicles are clearly seen within it.

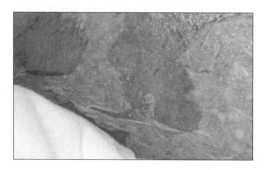

Fig. 1.110 Staphylococcal scalded skin syndrome
The organism, usually in an area of impetigo, releases 'exfoliatin' — a toxin which causes a split to occur high in the epidermis so that large areas become loosened (see also Fig. 8.27).

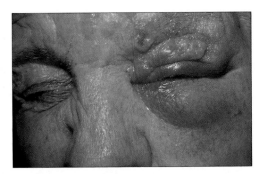

Fig. 1.111 Herpes zoster
Grouped vesicles are seen within the territory of the ophthalmic division of the trigeminal nerve. The absence of vesicles on the side of the nose implies that the naso-ciliary branch was not involved. For this reason, despite the inflammation and oedema of the eyelids, the cornea itself was not affected.

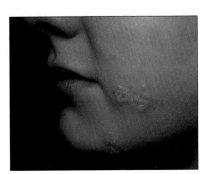

Fig. 1.112 Herpes Simplex Infections
Recurrent herpes simplex
This episode of herpes simplex was triggered by excessive sun exposure during a skiing holiday. Vesicles in the upper group of lesions are becoming pustular; the lower group has reached the crusting stage.

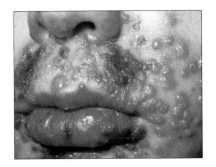

Fig. 1.113 Eczema herpeticum
This patient with atopic eczema had an unusually widespread herpes simplex infection of the face, but remained well and cleared quickly with oral acyclovir. Thereafter he avoided being kissed by his mother when she had an active cold sore.

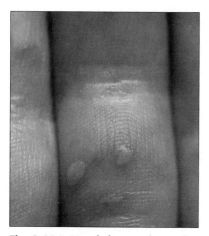

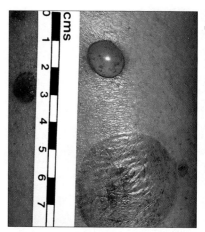

Fig. 1.114 Hand, foot and mouth disease
The small greyish vesicles, with a faint pink rim, are typical of this Coxsackie infection. The patient suffered from a short spell of fever and malaise but her children, with similar skin lesions, remained well.

Fig. 1.115 Bullous insect bite reaction
These blisters are large and under pressure; some also contain blood. These are features of blisters arising from underneath the epidermis rather than within it. Insect bites are particularly liable to become bullous on the legs.

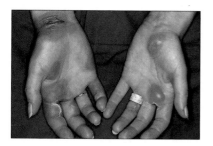

Fig. 1.116 Fixed drug eruption
This unusually severe bullous reaction was due to a barbiturate tablet and recurred each time one was taken.

PUSTULES

The presence of pus does not automatically imply bacterial infection. **Pustular psoriasis**, for example, localized (Fig. 1.117) or generalized (Figs. 1.118 and 1.119), has no infective component. Nor has **pyoderma gangrenosum** (Figs. 1.120 and 1.121), the main associations of which are with ulcerative colitis, Crohn's disease, polyarthritis (Fig. 1.122), a monoclonal gammopathy, or leukaemia. Even the obvious pustules of **acne** (Figs. 5.20 and 5.27) and **rosacea** (Fig. 1.26) have no straight-forward infective cause.

However, many pustular eruptions, particularly of the hair follicles, do have a bacterial (Figs. 1.123 and 1.124) or fungal (Fig. 1.125) cause. **Pityrosporum folliculitis** of the trunk, for example (Fig.3.10), is due to the overgrowth of commensal yeasts. In addition the blisters of some **viral infections**, for example, herpes simplex (Fig.1.112), herpes zoster (Fig. 1.111) and chicken pox, pass typically through a pustular phase. The lesions of chronic **gonococcal septicaemia** may become pustular too (Fig. 1.126) as may eczematous vesicles.

Other blisters may contain pus, as in **subcorneal pustular dermatosis** which may be associated with an underlying gammopathy. Occasionally pustular eruptions are **drug induced** for example by halides or frusemide.

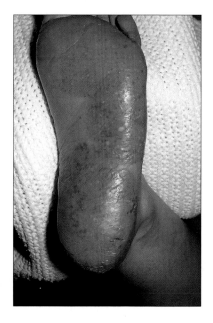

Fig. 1.117 Localized pustular psoriasis (palmo-plantar pustulosis)
Sharply demarcated erythema studded with pustules and their brown scaly remnants.

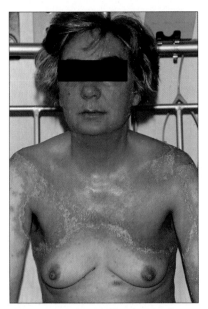

Fig. 1.118 Generalized pustular psoriasis
This patient had suffered for many years from episodes in which waves of erythema, bounded by areas of sterile pustulation, spread centrifugally across her skin. The appearance was very different from that of ordinary psoriasis, and these attacks were accompanied by malaise, fever and a leucocytosis.

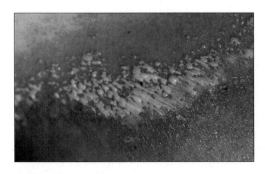

Fig. 1.119 Generalized pustular psoriasis
The pustules of acute generalized pustular psoriasis are sterile and arise on a background of erythema. Trigger factors include the sudden cessation of systemic or highly potent topical corticosteroid therapy.

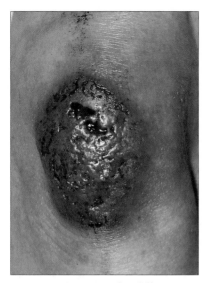

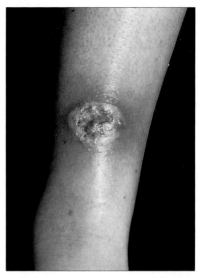

Figs. 1.120–1.122 The different faces of pyoderma gangrenosum
1.120 This massive inflammatory swelling is beginning to discharge pus through a number of small openings (cribriform).

1.121 The classical appearance of a polycyclic purulent ulcer with an inflamed edge — the association here was with ulcerative colitis. Other possible causes include Crohn's disease, rheumatoid arthritis and paraproteinaemia.

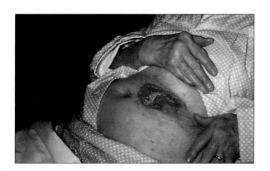

1.122 This longstanding abdominal ulcer was due to pyoderma gangrenosum, a rare complication of rheumatoid arthritis.

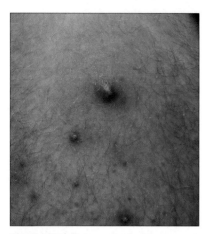

Fig. 1.123 Furunculosis Always check for diabetes, even though the chances of finding it are slim. It is more rewarding to swab the carrier sites of the patient and contacts for staphylococci.

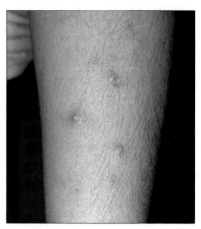

Fig. 1.124 Papulo-necrotic tuberculide
These apparently trivial pustules drew attention to an important tuberculous lymphadenitis.

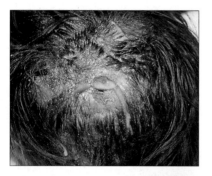

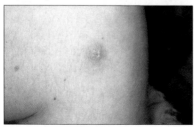

Fig. 1.125 Scalp ringworm
This degree of pustulation suggests a fungus derived from an animal source. Those that spread from human to human usually cause much less inflammation. Trichophyton verrucosum (the organism causing cattle ringworm) was later isolated from the area. The diagnosis became obvious to his family doctor only after several courses of anti-biotics proved ineffective. A small area of scarred alopecia remained after antifungal treatment was completed.

Fig. 1.126 Gonococcal septic emboli
Crops of unspectacular pustules in the skin secondary to pelvic sepsis.

CYSTS

Skin cysts are common, usually single, and an isolated finding. Straightforward examples include **epidermoid cysts** (Fig. 1.127) and **pilar cysts** (both once known as sebaceous cysts) and **milial cysts** (Figs. 1.128 and 1.129). Multiple epidermoid cysts are a feature of **Gardner's syndrome** (with polyposis of the colon) and of **Gorlin's syndrome** (with multiple naevoid basal cell carcinomas (Fig. 1.70)). The multiple cysts of **steatocystoma multiplex** (Fig. 1.130) contain oily sebum and are inherited as an autosomal dominant trait. Degenerative **myxoid cysts** (Figs. 1.131 and 4.77) occur near the proximal nail folds and may groove the nail. Cysts are also part of severe **acne** (Fig. 1.132), the diagnosis being made easy by the surrounding lesions.

Cysts may also arise as developmental anomalies. **Pre-auricular cysts** (Fig.1.136) or sinuses are found in the Treacher–Collins and Goldenhar syndromes. **Branchial cysts** are painless swellings in the upper neck; **thyroglossal cysts** lie in the midline of the neck and move when the tongue does; **congenital dermoid cysts**, especially common near the outer third of the eyebrow and on the nose, may have an opening from which hairs protrude (Fig. 1.133).

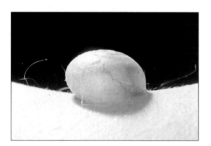

Fig. 1.127 Epidermoid cyst
An unusually protruberant example which has a central punctum and is filled with cheesy material.

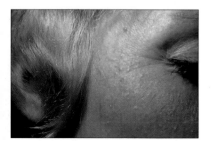

Fig. 1.128 Milia
Multiple tiny milia on the cheek of a young woman, apparently arising after sunburn.

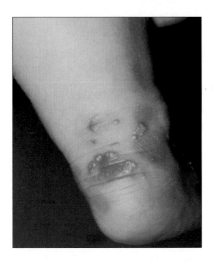

Fig. 1.129 Milia
Grouped milia often follow subepidermal blistering, as seen here in a child with dystrophic epidermolysis bullosa. Similar changes may be seen in porphyria cutanea tarda.

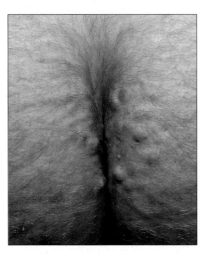

Fig. 1.130 Steatocystoma multiplex
These multiple yellowish cysts contained oily sebum and here were inherited as an autosomal dominant trait with no associated features.

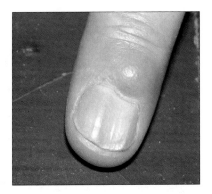

Fig. 1.131 Myxoid cyst
This is not koilonychia. Pressure from a
long-standing, jelly-filled cyst was
responsible for the grooved nail plate (see
also Fig. 4.77).

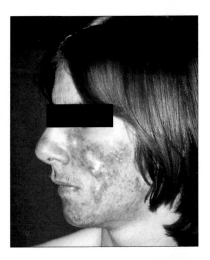

Fig. 1.132 Cystic acne
Patient needed systemic retinoid
treatment.

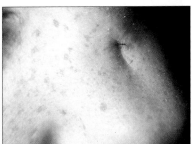

Fig. 1.133 Congenital dermoid cyst
A tuft of hairs arising from a pit on a
broadened nasal bridge. Removal is
always difficult and should be performed
by a specialist.

SINUSES

Persistent suppuration may be due to an underlying sinus. Suspicion should be raised by an intermittent purulent discharge from the chin or submental area (**dental sinus** (Fig. 1.134) or an underlying **osteomyelitis** (Fig. 1.135)), in front of the ear (**pre-auricular cysts and sinuses** (Fig. 1.136)), the lower third of the neck in front of the sternomastoid muscle (**branchial sinuses** or **scrofuloderma**), the lower mid-back (**spina bifida**), the sacrococcygeal region, the axillae, perineum and inguinal folds (**suppurative hidradenitis** (Fig. 1.137)), and the lower abdomen and perineum (**Crohn's disease** (Fig. 4.84)).

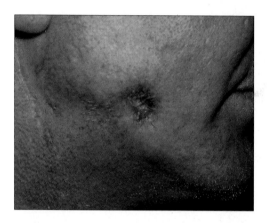

Fig. 1.134 Dental sinus
Neglect of oral hygiene led first to dental caries and later to an apical abscess which tracked outwards through the skin. Neither the patient nor his family doctor had realised that this was the cause of the intermittent bouts of swelling and discharge of foul-smelling material. The pouting sinus opening is typically surrounded by a sunken area. Treatment should be directed to the tooth and not the skin.

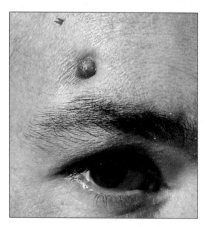

Fig. 1.135 Osteomyelitis of frontal bone
This little granuloma appeared innocuous but overlay an area of osteomyelitis of the frontal bone with which it communicated via a sinus.

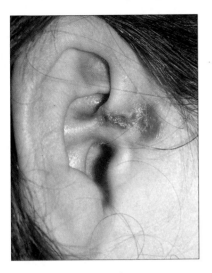

Fig. 1.136 Preauricular cysts and sinuses

This patient had a purulent discharge at the classic site, just in front of the ascending limb of the helix. These cysts or pits are often asymptomatic and bilateral. The sinus tract may blend with the periosteum of the auditory canal. Associated developmental abnormalities of the branchial apparatus may coexist.

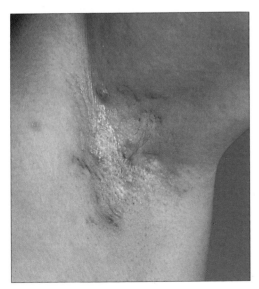

Fig. 1.137 Suppurative hidradenitis

A suppurative inflammation of apocrine glands in the armpits and groins — may be associated with acne. The armpit shows scars, chronically discharging sinuses and an inflammatory nodule forming superiorly.

Chapter 2

Shapes

Individual lesions may themselves take up a particular shape; alternatively, separate lesions may arrange themselves into a characteristic configuration. Terms like 'annular', can therefore be applied to individual lesions or to their groupings.

ANNULAR

Annular lesions are common and arise in many ways, ranging from the centrifugal expansion of a focus of infection to ill-understood immunological processes. Some are diagnostic and several signal internal disorders.

The hallmark of **urticaria** (Figs. 1.32–1.34) is its transience; annular wheals seldom last for more than a day. **Figurate erythemas** (Figs. 2.1–2.6), on the other hand, tend to be chronic, with serpiginous and erythematous rings which expand slowly and come and go over many weeks. Possible causes include internal malignancy, connective tissue disorders, drug sensitivity, bacterial, fungal or yeast infections, rheumatic heart disease and worm infestations. More often no cause is found.

The annular lesions of **erythema chronicum migrans** follow a tick bite (Figs. 2.7 and 2.8) and are due to the spirochaete Borrelia burgdorferi. An erythematous ring, or occasionally more than one, expands slowly and may reach over 20cm in diameter. The skin changes may usher in other manifestations including arthritis, arrhythmia, meningitis and cranial nerve palsies.

As its name implies, the erythematous lesions of **erythema multiforme** vary in their appearance and ring or target-like ones are common (Fig. 1.12). Herpes simplex is the most common trigger, but it may also follow other viral (e.g. orf or hepatitis), mycoplasma, bacterial or fungal infections. Rarely it draws attention to an underlying malignancy or is a reaction to radiotherapy. Some drugs (e.g. sulphonamides) may also provoke an attack.

The skin coloured lesions of **granuloma annulare** are most common on the backs of the hands (Fig. 2.9) or on the sides of children's fingers. The rings expand slowly but few reach more than 2cm in diameter. Multiple lesions tend to be papular rather than ring-like and may be a warning of underlying diabetes mellitus. Purple indurated rings merit a biopsy to exclude cutaneous **sarcoidosis** (Fig. 2.10) which itself has numerous patterns of internal involvement. Indurated, pink scaly annular plaques are seen in tuberculoid and borderline **tuberculoid leprosy**. The central parts of these rings are pale and anaesthetic (Figs. 1.53, 9.8 and 9.9). Biopsy helps to confirm the diagnosis.

Other causes of rings include **psoriasis** (Figs. 2.11 and 2.12), **pityriasis rosea** (Fig. 2.13), **fungal infections** (Figs. 2.14 and 2.15), **syphilis** (Figs. 2.16 and 2.17), **basal cell carcinoma** (Fig. 1.63 and 1.64), **perforating elastoma** (Fig. 2.18) and **linear IgA disease** (Fig. 2.19). Occasionally **mycosis fungoides**, a cutaneous T cell lymphoma, presents with irregular erythematous and scaly rings (Fig. 1.75).

Figs. 2.1–2.6 Annular erythema

This is a convenient descriptive term for a number of, probably unrelated, clinical entities.

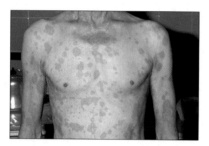

2.1 Widespread blotchy erythema with some annular features which appeared transiently as a result of a reaction to systemic penicillin treatment.

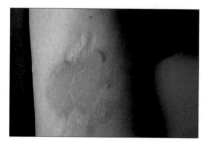

2.2 A striking erythematous ring which enlarged slowly, trailing an inner rim of scaling. The lesion lasted for a few weeks before fading and no internal cause was found.

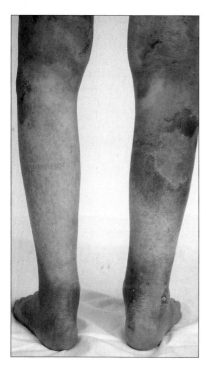

2.3 These annular lesions were part of the glucagonoma syndrome. The patient had an islet cell carcinoma of the pancreas. The annular lesions in some areas showed a superficial necrotic rim and moved slowly across the skin. Other features included diabetes, iron deficiency and a shiny red tongue (Fig. 4.47).

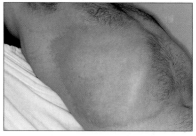

2.4 This patient had a carcinoma at the lower end of the oesophagus. A massive area of annular erythema persisted for many weeks on the side of the chest and was thought to be a response to the tumour.

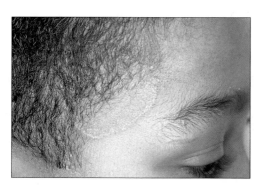

2.5 In this lesion on the temple, the trailing edge of peeling is still obvious but the annular ring itself has now virtually faded. No underlying cause was ever found for this eruption which came and went over a period of a few months.

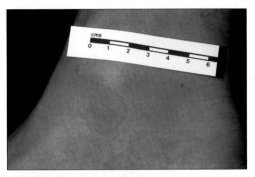

2.6 This fleeting erythematous ring on the ankle lasted for just 24h. An association here with rheumatic fever allowed the condition to be called erythema marginatum.

Figs. 2.7–2.8 Lyme disease

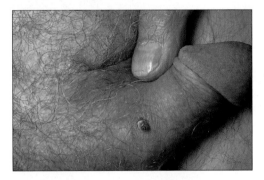

2.7 The spirochaete causing this condition is transmitted to man via tick bites. Here a tick is seen attached to the shaft of the penis.

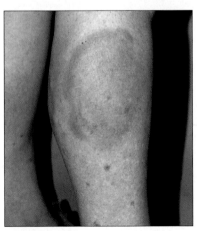

2.8 This annular lesion on the calf (erythema chronicum migrans) appeared some ten days after a tick bite and enlarged slowly. The eruption responded well to amoxycillin treatment and the patient had no arthritis, neurological involvement, or myocarditis.

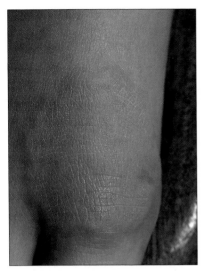

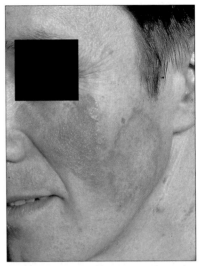

Fig. 2.9 Granuloma annulare
A typical plaque on the back of one knuckle. As is usually the case, diabetes was not present.

Fig. 2.10 Sarcoidosis
Annular lesions are particularly common in sarcoidosis of the face and neck. The rim of the lesions has a brownish tinge, characteristic of a granuloma.

Fig. 2.11–2.12 Psoriasis

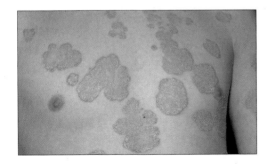

2.11 Psoriasis is often annular; sometimes because treatment is concentrated on the centre of lesions and sometimes for no obvious reason. In this example, the centre of the patch above the nipple is now clearing to form a ring-like lesion, the other plaques already show raised active rims.

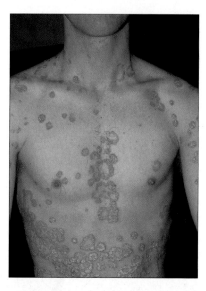

2.12 The annular lesions on the sternum and neck contrast with the straight-forward plaques on the upper abdomen.

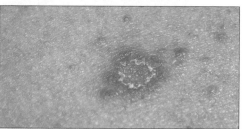

Fig. 2.13 Pityriasis rosea
The small oval patches of pityriasis rosea show a characteristic rim of scaling inside the edge of the lesion.

Figs. 2.14–2.15 Ringworm infections

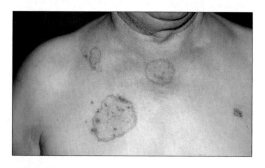

2.14 Scrapings from the active edge of these rings on the front of the chest yielded a dermatophyte fungus on culture. The infection had been picked up from his newly acquired puppy.

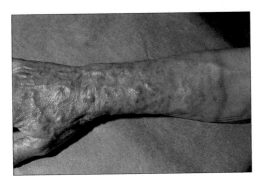

2.15 Tinea incognito. If a topical steroid preparation is mistakenly used to treat ringworm, the morphology quickly changes and the diagnosis becomes difficult. In this case the rim of the lesion is seen half way up the forearm. The involved skin of the lower forearm and hand shows atrophy and follicular papules due to the fungus.

Fig. 2.16–2.17 Syphilis

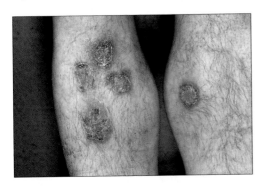

2.16 Syphilis remains a great mimic. These lesions, somewhat reminiscent of discoid eczema, were a secondary syphilide of annular type.

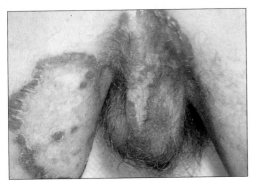

2.17 Tinea cruris is being mimicked; however, annular and arcuate lesions are also typical of the nodular form of late syphilis.

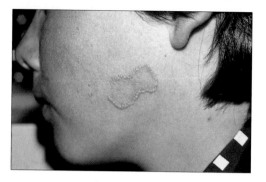

Fig. 2.18 Perforating elastoma

Elastic tissue is being extruded through the epidermis at the rough bumpy border of this lesion. Important systemic associations include penicillamine therapy, Down's syndrome, Marfan's syndrome, osteogenesis imperfecta, the Ehlers-Danlos syndrome and pseudoxanthoma elasticum.

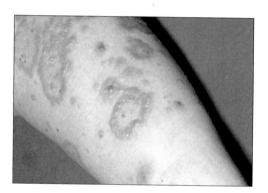

Fig. 2.19 Chronic bullous dermatosis of childhood

Rings of vesicles, looking rather like pearls strung together as a necklace, are common in this self-limiting disorder. The presence of a band of IgA at the basement membrane explains its other name — linear IgA disease. An associated enteropathy, as in the case of dermatitis herpetiformis, is seldom found.

BUTTERFLY

Eruptions on the cheeks, linked via the bridge of the nose, assume the shape of a butterfly, or a bat's wing. Systemic **lupus erythematosus** (Fig. 2.20), **pemphigus erythematosus** (Fig. 2.21), **rosacea** (Fig. 1.26) and **seborrhoeic dermatitis** (Fig. 1.17) may do this.

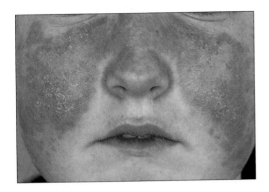

Fig. 2.20 Lupus erythematosus
The butterfly wing appearance can be seen both in systemic and in discoid lupus erythematosus. In the latter, as seen here, scaling and fixity of the lesions are important features.

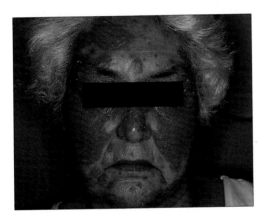

Fig. 2.21 Pemphigus erythematosus
A butterfly distribution can occur in conditions other than lupus erythematosus. These lesions start as thin roofed blisters and quickly become erosions.

LINEAR

TEMPORARY

Usually these have an obvious external cause. The burrows of **scabies** are linear (Fig. 2.22), as are the tracks of **larva migrans** (Fig. 2.23). **Mycobacterial** and **deep fungal infections** may cause nodules and ulcers lying along the line of lymphatic drainage (Fig. 2.24 and 2.25). **Insect bites** can be arranged in lines determined by clothing (Fig. 2.26). **Scratching** may leave linear excoriations or the linear wheals of dermographism (Fig. 2.27 and 1.34). Perhaps the 'flagellate erythema' of some bleomycin reactions is also based on scratching — the linearity of some cases of **dermatitis artefacta** certainly is (Fig. 2.28).

Warts can be seeded in lines along scratch marks; lines of psoriasis (Fig. 2.29) or lichen planus will also have followed scratches or cuts (by the Koebner phenomenon).

Corrosive liquids cause linear burns, a good clue to dermatitis artefacta. Similarly, photosensitizing **perfumes** can trickle across the skin leaving hyperpigmented lines (**Berloque dermatitis**) (Fig. 8.15). Linear erythema and then pigmentation may follow contact with **photosensitizing plants** (Fig. 2.30); and contact allergic dermatitis, due to plants such as primulae brushing against the skin, is also characteristically streaky (Fig. 2.31). Linear **contact dermatitis** may mimic the shape of the object which caused it, for example a hat band (Fig. 2.32), or a catheter (Fig. 2.33).

LONGSTANDING

Perhaps the most interesting are those that follow **Blaschko's** lines (Fig. 2.34). They are examples of cutaneous mosaicism and the lines represent the developmental movement of clones of cells. Mosaics have at least two cell populations which differ in one of several ways. In **incontinentia pigmenti** (Fig. 10.5) and **focal dermal hypoplasia**, the lines represent areas where the abnormal X chromosome was active. Chromosomal mosaicism may also lead to linear dyspigmentation. Some autosomal dominant traits occur in a mosaic form, leading, for example, to linear **Darier's disease** or **porokeratosis**. Linear **epidermal** (Fig. 2.35) or **sebaceous naevi** (Fig. 2.36) are presumably due to clones of cells which have undergone somatic mutation.

Lines of **psoriasis** or **lichen planus** along Blaschko's lines may be due to clones of cells especially susceptible to these conditions. Some believe that linear inflammatory naevi (Fig. 2.37) are linear eczema manifesting only in a clone of susceptible cells.

Other lines are due to other causes. Stretch marks reflect lines of skin tension (Fig. 2.38), as do some spontaneously occurring **keloids** (Fig. 8.9). The linearity of some other lesions, such as *coup-de-sabre* **morphoea** (Fig. 2.39), macular **amyloid** (Fig. 2.40) and **dermatomyositis** (Fig. 2.41), still lacks explanation.

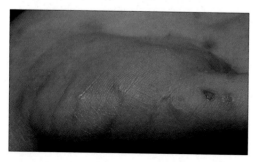

Fig. 2.22 Scabies burrows
Side-lighting helps to show up the slightly raised curved burrows on the thenar eminence. The acarus will lie at the most recent, least scaly end of a burrow.

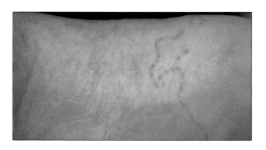

Fig. 2.23 Larva migrans (creeping eruption)
Six weeks after a holiday in the tropics an itchy red line began to move slowly and tortuously across his instep. It was the track of a hookworm larva, picked up from contact with dog faeces on a beach.

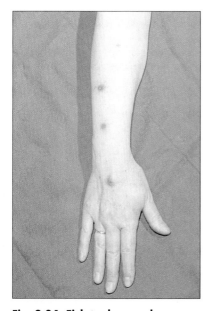

Fig. 2.24 Fish tank granuloma
This tropical fish fancier acquired an infection with Mycobacterium marinum on the back of one hand while cleaning out her aquarium. The nodules which appeared later on her forearm lay along the line of lymphatic drainage. This type of spread is referred to as sporotrichoid, being even more striking in sporotrichosis itself.

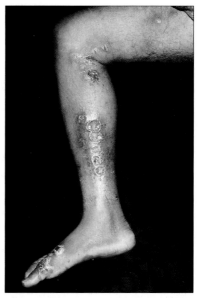

Fig. 2.25 Sporotrichosis
The disease is common in tropical areas. The pathogen, sporothrix schenkii, penetrated the skin via a wound in the foot and extended up the leg along the line of the lymphatics, causing a linear array of ulcerated nodules.

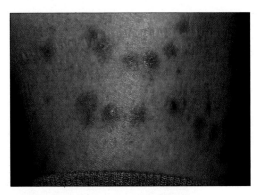

Fig. 2.26 Insect bites
Socks tend to slip down. The upper level of this grey sock varied from the highest postion, shown here by the linear indentation made by its elastic top, to the lower one depicted. Two distinct lines of bites are visible — their positions being determined by intermediate sock top levels. They have been scratched and are now purpuric.

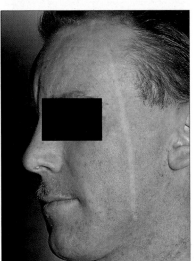

Fig. 2.27 White dermographism
This is a white reaction (cf. red dermographism, Fig. 1.34) to stroking or scratching the skin. It is seen most often, but not always, in atopic patients.

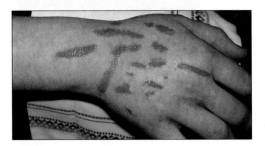

Fig. 2.28 Dermatitis artefacta
No-one ever found out precisely how this girl created the linear lesions on the back of her hand, but the diagnosis of dermatitis artefacta was never in doubt. Linearity is often a useful clue in this condition.

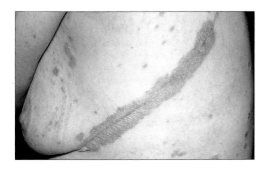

Fig. 2.29 Linear psoriasis
This patient with longstanding active psoriasis recovered well from her chest operation but three weeks later psoriasis appeared along the line of the scar. This is the Koebner (isomorphic) phenomenon, also seen in lichen planus. It may be helpful diagnostically.

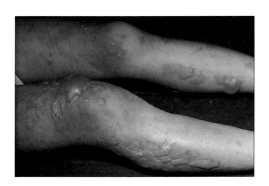

**Fig. 2.30
Phytophotodermatitis**
The giant hogweed plant contains photosensitizing psoralens which are transferred to the skin by direct contact. Subsequent exposure to sunlight causes redness and blistering.

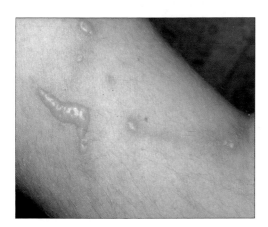

Fig. 2.31 Plant contact dermatitis
Primula plants are common sensitizers. The act of brushing against primula leaves was enough to cause this characteristic mixture of itchy red lines and linear blisters on a highly allergic patient's arm.

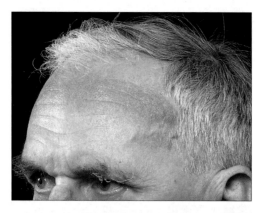

Fig. 2.32 Allergic contact dermatitis

This patient knew that he had been sensitized to chrome, present in cement, during his time in the building industry. However, he did not realise that his hat-band was made of leather tanned with chromate and that chrome allergy was also responsible for the line of chronic pigmented contact dermatitis across his forehead.

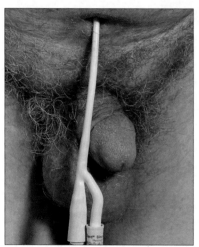

Fig. 2.33 Contact dermatitis

Wherever this catheter touched the skin it caused a line of contact dermatitis.

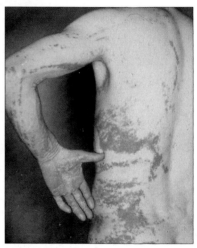

Fig. 2.34 The epidermal naevus syndrome

This bizarre pattern, made up of lines of reddish warty lesions had been present only on the left side since birth. Blaschko described these characteristic lines in 1901 and they are now known to be a feature of cutaneous mosaicism. A variety of skeletal, neurological and ocular abnormalities may also be found in the epidermal naevus syndrome.

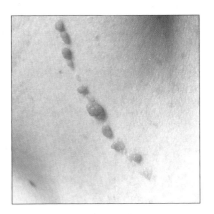

Fig. 2.35 Linear epidermal naevus
Unlike warts, these lesions are present
from birth and tend to follow Blaschko's
lines.

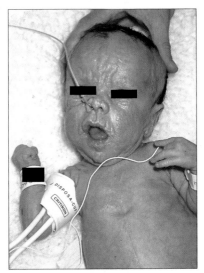

**Fig. 2.36 Unilateral epidermal
naevus**
This extensive linear naevus of sebaceous
type followed Blaschko's lines and was
associated with many other congenital
defects.

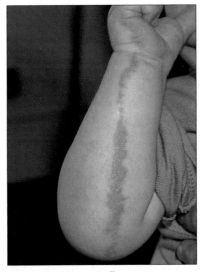

**Fig. 2.37 Linear inflammatory
naevus**
This itchy linear naevus, present at birth,
failed to clear up with topical steroids.

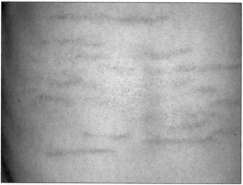

Fig. 2.38 Striae distensae

The stretch marks on the back were due to growth spurts in an adolescent. Initially bluish-red, later they became white and atrophic. The common abdominal striae of pregnancy look similar. Other causes: rapid weight gain and excessive corticosteroids (Cushing's disease, local and systemic steroid treatment).

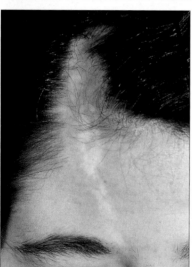

Fig. 2.39 Morphoea — en coup de sabre

There is a linear depression from the eyebrow to the scalp due to localized scleroderma plus atrophy of the underlying bone. Facial hemiatrophy may be a complication.

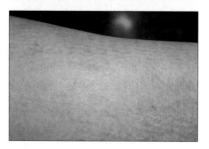

Fig. 2.40 Macular amyloid

The linear and rippled appearance of the pigmentation is typical. The condition is most common in people from Asia, the Middle East and South America. Lesions are itchy but without systemic accompaniments.

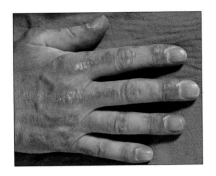

Fig. 2.41 Dermatomyositis
This 55 year old patient had an underlying lung cancer. The papules over the knuckles (Gottron's papules) and the erythematous proximal nail folds are highly characteristic; so too are the lines of erythema on the backs of the fingers and over the extensor tendons on the back of the hand (Dowling's lines).

RETICULATE (NET-LIKE)

Livedo reticularis (Fig. 2.42) is an important physical sign, which may have systemic associations such as with cerebrovascular disease (**Sneddon's syndrome**). Many patients with this association also have raised **anticardiolipin** antibodies and/or **lupus anticoagulant**; some have underlying systemic **lupus erythematosus**. Other possible systemic associations include **polyarteritis nodosa** (Fig. 2.43) and **cryoglobulinaemia**. A similar pattern of mottled discoloration is seen in **erythema ab igne** (Fig. 2.44), itself sometimes a clue to hypothyroidism. **Poikiloderma vasculare atrophicans** (Fig. 2.45) and **paraneoplastic reticulate pigmentation** (Fig. 2.46) are rare.

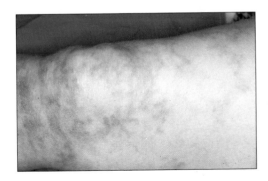

Fig. 2.42 Livedo reticularis
Fixed, purplish and reticulate; look for other evidence of lupus erythematosus, polyarteritis nodosa and the antiphospholipid syndrome with its high risk of cerebrovascular disease and deep vein thrombosis.

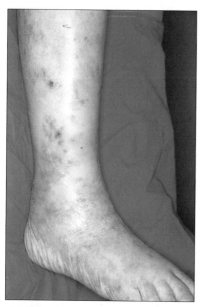

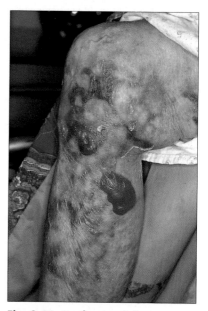

Fig. 2.43 Cutaneous polyarteritis nodosa
The skin signs consist of painful papules and nodules together with a background of ill-defined livedo reticularis. No systemic evidence of polyarteritis was found in this patient.

Fig. 2.44 Erythema ab igne
A patient with hypothyroidism who liked to sit too near the fire. These blisters represent a burn arising on a background of chronic thermal damage.

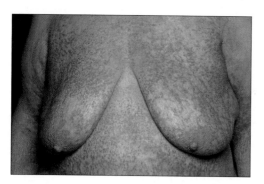

Fig. 2.45 Poikiloderma vasculare atrophicans
This characteristic mixture of atrophy, pigmentation and telangiectasia is one of the several cutaneous eruptions which can eventually turn into a cutaneous T cell lymphoma.

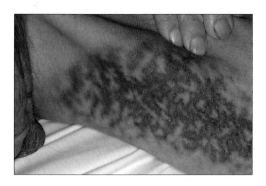

Fig. 2.46 Paraneoplastic pigmentation
Seen in an unusual position on the inner aspect of one thigh. The lesions became heavily pigmented during the development of a carcinoma of the stomach.

UMBILICATED

The lesions of **molluscum contagiosum** (Fig. 2.47) are umbilicated: a white core can be squeezed out through the central opening. The old name for a **keratoacanthoma** (Fig. 2.48) was 'molluscum sebaceum'. It too has a central keratotic plug surrounded by a fleshy base. Finally, lesions seen in the pustular phase of some **viral infections**, for example in chickenpox and herpes simplex (Fig. 2.49), can be umbilicated.

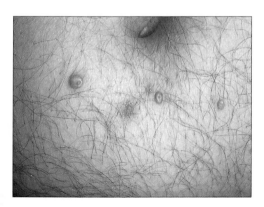

Fig. 2.47 Molluscum contagiosum
A typical scattering of small domed shiny lesions with a central umbilicated pore.

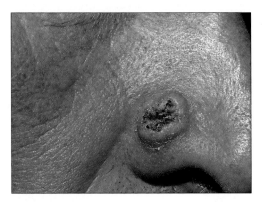

**Fig. 2.48
Keratoacanthoma**
These come up quickly, over a
few weeks, and their histology
is close to that of a squamous
cell carcinoma. The central
keratotic plug and fleshy rim
are typical of a
keratoacanthoma which, if left
alone for long enough, would
disappear spontaneously.

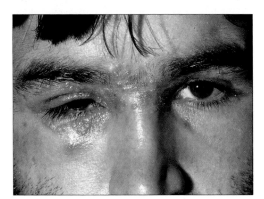

**Fig. 2.49 Eczema
herpeticum**
The umbilicated vesicles were
the main clue to diagnosis in
this patient with long-standing
atopic eczema.

Chapter 3

Distributions

Skin disorders can be localized or generalized, or follow a particular distribution. This offers a third important clue to diagnosis, to be added to the information provided by a close examination of the primary lesions and their configuration.

EXTENSOR

Some rashes have a predilection for extensor surfaces, sometimes encouraged by trauma. Hyperkeratosis, for example, is seen on the knees of those who kneel at work or at prayer. **Psoriasis** and **pityriasis rubra pilaris** (Fig. 3.1) also favour the elbows, knees and extensor aspects of the limbs.

The extensor distribution of the small excoriated groups of blisters in **dermatitis herpetiformis** (Figs. 1.107, 1.108 and 3.25) helps to differentiate it clinically from **pemphigoid** (Fig. 1.106). The purpuric lesions of small vessel vasculitis, especially of **Henoch–Schönlein purpura** (Fig. 1.41) also favour extensor sites.

Tuberous xanthomas (Fig. 3.2) are seen on pressure areas such as the elbows, knees and extensor aspects of the limbs. They are associated with hyperlipidaemia. Finally, atrophic scarring and blistering of the knees and elbows are common in the dystrophic types of **epidermolysis bullosa** (Figs. 1.101–1-102).

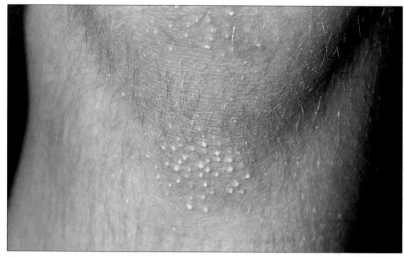

Fig. 3.1 Pityriasis rubra pilaris
Of the many clinical patterns, this is perhaps the mildest. In the familial variety, the follicular hyperkeratoses are largely confined to the points of the elbows and knees. Vitamin deficiency is not a factor.

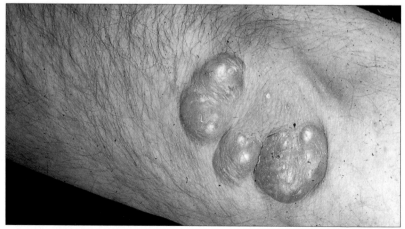

Fig. 3.2 Tuberous xanthomas
The extensor distribution and yellowish colour suggest the diagnosis. In this case an abnormal serum lipoprotein profile was found.

FLEXURAL

The armpits and groin and the skin under the breasts carry their own range of skin disorders. Many are infective as opportunistic organisms flourish under warm moist conditions, particularly in the obese. Diphtheroid overgrowth causes **erythrasma** (Fig. 3.3) to which diabetics are especially prone, as they are to **candidal intertrigo** (Fig. 3.4). An overgrowth of commensal yeasts contributes to the development of **seborrhoeic eczema** in the flexures (Fig. 3.5). Friction and infection are important in the flexural localization of chronic benign familial pemphigus (**Hailey–Hailey disease**). Yellow axillary sweat may be due to the overgrowth of pigment-producing diphtheroids on the axillary hairs (**trichomycosis axillaris** (Fig. 9.19)).

The armpits and groins also contain apocrine glands, important in the abscesses and sinuses of **suppurative hidradenitis** (Fig. 1.137), which may itself be confused with cutaneous Crohn's disease. Inflammation of the apocrine glands also occurs in the itchy papules of **Fox–Fordyce disease**.

Finally, many dermatoses look different in the flexures. **Psoriasis**, for example, tends to be smooth there, rather than scaly (Fig. 3.6). Clothing **contact dermatitis** affects the rim of the axilla but spares its vault, in contrast to seborrhoeic eczema or allergic reactions to deodorants.

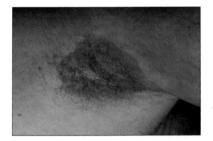

Fig. 3.3 Erythrasma
Well demarcated, reddish-brown, often finely wrinkled or scaly areas in the flexures may be due to this. Look for the pink fluorescence under Wood's light which is typical of this diphtheroid overgrowth. There is sometimes an association with diabetes mellitus.

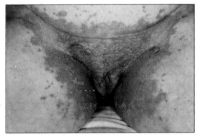

Fig. 3.4 Candida of the groin
Moist glazed areas of erythema, with soggy scaling and outlying satellite vesico-pustules. Diabetes mellitus was the predisposing cause here.

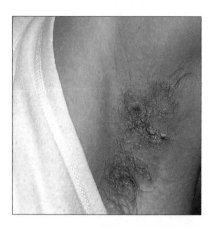

Fig. 3.5 Seborrhoeic eczema
Persistent red crusty areas in the armpits.

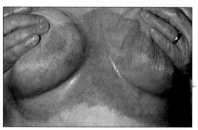

Fig. 3.6 Flexural psoriasis
The strong red colour and sharp
margination persist, but these areas are
shiny and smooth rather than obviously
scaly.Reproduced with permission from
Edwards, Bouchier, Haslett et al (eds),
Davidson's Principles and Practice of
Medicine, 17th edn., 1995, Churchill-
Livingstone, Edinburgh.

FOLLICULAR

Involvement of the hair follicles is a striking feature of some skin conditions.
Keratosis pilaris (Fig. 3.7), a common and harmless genodermatosis, is a good
example. Keratin plugs block the hair follicles on the outer arms and thighs. Some
varieties lead on to hair loss, especially of the eyebrows (ulerythema ophryogenes).

Follicular hyperkeratotic papules are a constant feature of early **pityriasis rubra
pilaris** (Figs. 3.1 and 5.8); later they are engulfed in a generalized redness and
scaliness. The idea that pityriasis rubra pilaris is due to vitamin A deficiency has
been disproved. Indeed follicular prominence of dietary origin (**phrynoderma**) is
not specific to vitamin A deficiency but follows a lack of several factors of which
vitamin A may be one. Follicular keratoses containing coiled hairs (Fig 3.8) may be
an early sign of **scurvy** and surrounded by perifollicular haemorrhages.

Occasionally **lichen planus** affects mainly the hair follicles, which then become spiny and keratotic (lichen plano-pilaris). Infiltration with mucin is responsible for the prominence of the hair follicles in **follicular mucinosis** (Fig. 4.21); a minority of cases are associated with a lymphoma.

In **perforating folliculitis** (Fig. 3.9), which may coexist with chronic renal disease or diabetes, keratotic follicular papules appear on the limbs. Follicular inflammation is seen in **pityrosporum folliculitis** (Fig. 3.10), in **bacterial folliculitis** (Fig. 1.123), and in **folliculitis decalvans** which is one cause of scarring alopecia. **Pseudomonas folliculitis** follows the use of a contaminated jacuzzi or hot tub. A chronic itchy folliculitis may be one skin manifestation of **HIV infection** (Fig. 3.11).

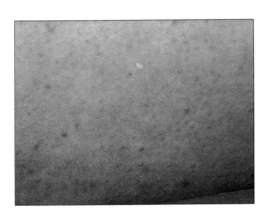

Fig. 3.7 Keratosis pilaris
A common and harmless genodermatosis — most marked on the outer aspects of the thighs and upper arms.

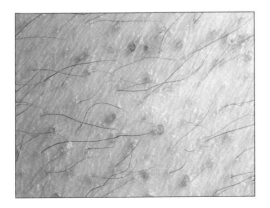

Fig. 3.8 Scurvy
Coiled hairs can be seen lying within plugged follicles. Later the follicles may become haemorrhagic.

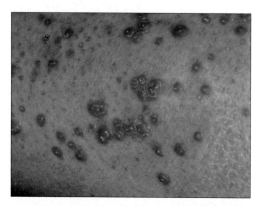

Fig. 3.9 Acquired perforating dermatosis
Aggregate groups of plugged and umbilicated papules: histology shows perforation into the dermis. Associated with chronic renal failure and/or diabetes.

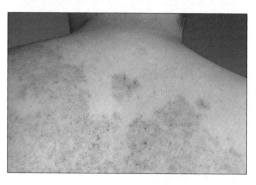

Fig. 3.10 Pityrosporum folliculitis
Overgrowth of commensal yeasts has led to this entity sometimes being called pityrosporum folliculitis. It may be seen in normal people, or in those with immunodeficiency, such as due to AIDS.

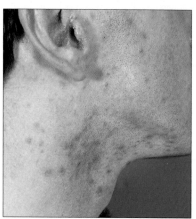

Fig. 3.11 Folliculitis and HIV infection
A stubborn mixture of seborrhoeic dermatitis (otitis externa) and itchy folliculitis was a useful pointer to the underlying HIV infection.

SEGMENTAL

A dermatomal pattern is determined by the distribution of nerves, not by the epidermal clones which create Blaschko's lines. **Capillary malformations**, for example, often seem to be arranged dermatomally (Figs. 3.12 and 3.13), and this fits the theory that their primary defect lies in the innervation of blood vessels. **Neurofibromatosis** (Fig. 3.23) and **vitiligo** (Fig. 3.14) can sometimes appear in a dermatomal configuration, which is also, of course, classically seen in **herpes zoster** (Figs. 3.15–3.18). **Telangiectases** are occasionally seen unilaterally (Fig. 3.19).

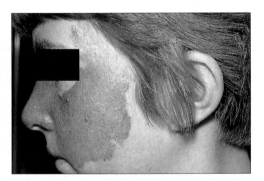

Fig. 3.12 Capillary malformation

Port wine stains often seem to be segmental. This shows an example largely confined to the maxillary branch of the trigeminal nerve.

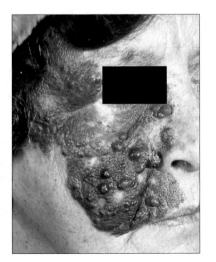

Fig. 3.13 Capillary malformation

The increasing nodularity which comes with age is well shown. Underlying involvement of the meninges and brain may lead to the Sturge-Weber syndrome. Capillary naevi on the limbs may be associated with arteriovenous shunts and limb hypertrophy.

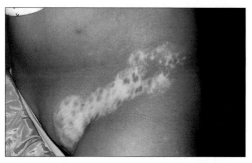

Fig. 3.14 Segmental vitiligo
In a young Asian girl. This type of vitiligo repigments more often than the generalized type.

Figs. 3.15–3.18 Herpes zoster

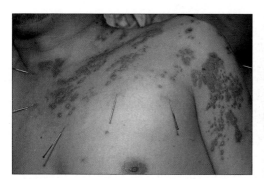

Fig. 3.15 The typical segmental lesions of herpes zoster over the shoulder. The grouped blisters are becoming pustular. The attempt at acupuncture had little effect.

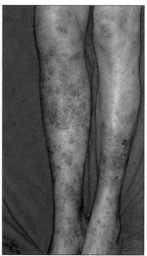

Fig. 3.16 Spread outside a single segment. In this patient, with chronic lymphatic leukaemia, the main segmental lesions were seen on the right leg, but the rest of the skin also showed a scattering of chickenpox-like lesions

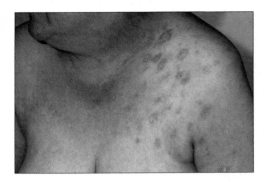

3.17 Motor involvement can occur. This patient had suffered from shingles in the C4 distribution, here shown by residual scarring.

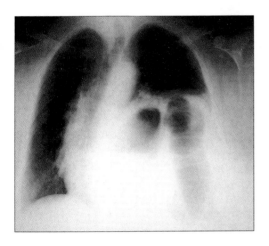

3.18 Involvement of the phrenic nerve led to diaphragmatic paralysis on that side.(Same patient as Fig. 3.17.)

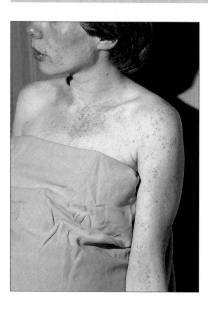

Fig. 3.19 Unilateral naevoid telangiectasia syndrome
Unilateral, segmental areas, showing numerous spider naevi, most commonly are seen in women, in connection with pregnancy and oestrogen medication. Occasionally they are seen in men with cirrhosis of the liver.

GROUPED

Sometimes grouping has an obvious exogenous cause such as with **insect bites** (Fig. 2.26). **Warts** (Fig. 5.40), **herpes simplex** (Fig. 3.20 and 3.21) and **zoster** (Fig. 3.15), **molluscum contagiosum** (Figs. 2.47 and 5.53) and **impetigo** are examples of infections which show grouping.

In **lymphangioma circumscriptum** (Fig. 3.22), the grouping of the lymph-filled blebs due to an abnormality of the underlying lymphatics, as is the occasional grouping of cutaneous **metastases** (Fig. 1.80).

Lesions may also be grouped because they arise from an underlying abnormality of nerve fibres, as in localized **neurofibromatosis** (Fig. 3.23) or of blood vessels, as in **unilateral naevoid telangiectasia** (Fig. 3.19) and **glomus tumours** (Fig. 3.24).

In **dermatitis herpetiformis**, groups of itchy vesicles occur on the elbows, shoulders, buttocks and on the scalp (Fig. 3.25).

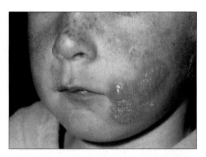

Fig. 3.20 Herpes simplex
The grouping of vesicles on an erythematous base is characteristic.

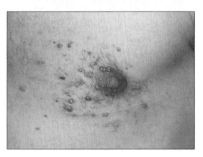

Fig. 3.21 Eczema herpeticum
Grouping is still apparent in this widespread and potentially serious complication of atopic eczema.

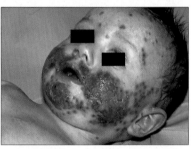

Fig. 3.22 Lymphangioma circumscriptum
Clusters of lymph-filled blebs, some of which also contain blood. Attempts to remove superficially (as here) are invariably followed by recurrence as the underlying abnormality is deep.

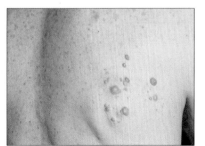

Fig. 3.23 Segmental neurofibromatosis
This probably represents a somatic mutation of the NF1 gene. The risk of an offspring developing full blown neurofibromatosis is not yet established.

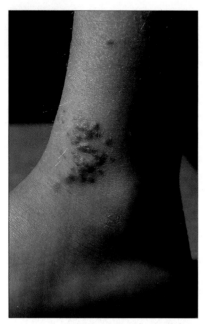

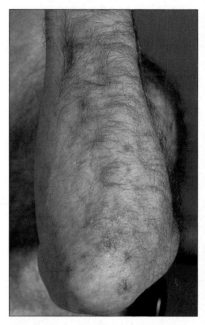

Fig. 3.24 Multiple glomus tumours
These are less painful than single lesions and may be inherited as an autosomal dominant trait.

Fig. 3.25 Dermatitis herpetiformis
The itchy blisters are characteristically grouped, most often on the elbows and knees, shoulder blades and sacrum. The association is with gluten enteropathy.

Chapter 4

Regions

The dermatology of some regions differs enough from that of the rest of the skin to need special mention.

HAIR

HAIR LOSS (ALOPECIA)

This has many patterns and many causes. Always decide on three points before making a diagnosis:

1. Does the skin in the bald areas show any evidence of a skin disease (e.g. redness, scaling, crusting or pustulation)? If so, consider **scalp ringworm** (Fig. 1.125), **lichen planus**, and **discoid lupus erythematosus** (Fig. 4.1).

2. Have the hair follicles been replaced by scar tissue? If so, follicular openings can no longer be seen through a lens. Consider scarring from **burns** (Fig. 4.2), **animal ringworm, carbuncles, radiodermatitis** (Fig. 8.52) or a **metastatic carcinoma** (Fig. 4.3). Possible skin causes include **follicular lichen planus, discoid lupus erythematosus** (Fig. 4.1), a cicatricial **basal cell carcinoma, necrobiosis** and **sarcoidosis. Alopecia areata** (Figs. 4.4 and 4.5) and **traction alopecia** (Fig. 4.6) are non-scarring.

3. Is the hair loss diffuse rather than localized? Causes of diffuse hair loss include **cytotoxic drugs** (Fig. 4.7) and **telogen effluvium** which occurs some three months after childbirth or a severe febrile illness. Other causes include **androgenic alopecia** (often diffuse in women (Fig. 4.8)), **iron deficiency** and **endocrine disorders** (e.g. hypo- or hyperthyroidism, hypopituitarism). In addition localized alopecia may eventually become generalized, as in **alopecia totalis**, though this should be distinguished from a congenital ectodermal defect such as **hypohidrotic ectodermal dysplasia** (Fig.7.1).

AN EXCESS OF HAIR

Hirsutism is a growth of coarse terminal hair in a male sexual pattern, but in a female or prepubertal child. Most cases are familial, racial, or post-menopausal, but the possibility of **virilization** must always be considered (Fig. 4.9 and 4.10). Causes include abnormalities of the ovaries (tumours or polycystic), adrenals (congenital adrenal hyperplasia, tumours, Cushing's syndrome) or pituitary (acromegaly, prolactinoma). Androgens and anabolic steroids have the same effect.

Hypertrichosis is an excess of hair in a non-sexual distribution (Figs. 4.11 and 4.12). It may be just in one area, such as the base of the spine in **spina bifida occulta** (Fig. 4.13), or over a **Becker's naevus** (Fig. 4.14). Localized hypertrichosis may also be found under a plaster cast or as a response to chronic irritation. Generalized hypertrichosis is part of several disorders including **porphyria** (Figs. 8.18 and 8.19), and some **mucopolysaccharidoses**. It is also a feature of **anorexia nervosa**, gross malnutrition and the **foetal alcohol syndrome**. Some drugs can cause it too, especially cyclosporin and minoxidil. Finally, and very rarely, generalized hypertrichosis can offer a clue to an **underlying neoplasm**.

ABNORMAL HAIR COLOUR

Premature greying is especially common in autoimmune disorders such as pernicious anaemia; it is also associated with premature ageing, e.g. in **Werner's syndrome** (Fig. 4.15).

A faint yellow tinge (Fig. 4.16) can be seen in the hairs of tyrosine-positive, but not tyrosine-negative **albinism**. Localized areas of white hair (**poliosis**, (Fig. 4.17)) occur in **Waardenburg's syndrome** (with heterochromia iridis, confluent eyebrows and deafness), in **piebaldism**, in the **Vogt-Koyanagi syndrome** (with bilateral uveitis), over areas of **vitiligo** and after the regrowth of **alopecia areata** in older people (Fig. 4.4).

Pale hair is a feature of untreated **phenylketonuria**, **Menkes syndrome**, the **Chediak-Higashi syndrome** and protein malnutrition (**kwashiorkor**). In the latter, alternating periods of good and bad nutrition cause darker and paler bands to appear in the hairs (the flag sign).

Some drugs alter hair colour. **Chloroquine** and **mephenesin**, for example, can lighten it; **minoxidil** and **diazoxide** can darken it. Some local applications stain the hair, for example **dithranol**.

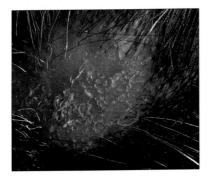

Fig. 4.1 Discoid lupus erythematosus
This lady's main worry was a bald patch at the front of her scalp. There is follicular plugging and scarring with minimal inflammation. Small lesions of discoid lupus erythematosus were also noted on her face (Fig. 2.20).

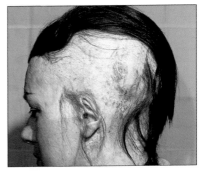

Fig. 4.2 Burn scar
This patient fell into a fire as a child burning her ear and thereafter needing a wig to cover her scarred scalp.

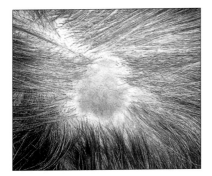

Fig. 4.3 Alopecia neoplastica
These flat pink hairless areas are due to secondary deposits from a carcinoma of the breast.

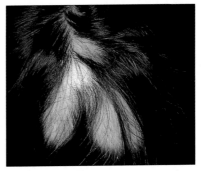

Fig. 4.4 Patchy alopecia areata
Early regrowth with pale hairs can be seen.

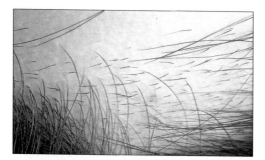

Fig. 4.5 Alopecia areata
'Exclamation-mark' hairs, broken off about 4mm from the scalp, and narrower proximally, are pathognomonic of alopecia areata.

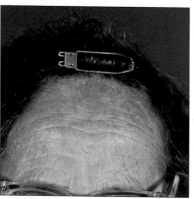

Fig. 4.6 Traction alopecia
Frontal alopecia in women is not always due to systemic lupus erythematosus. Longterm use of rollers can cause an impressive 'marginal' alopecia too.

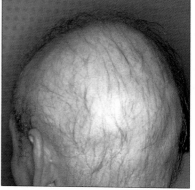

Fig. 4.7 Drug-induced alopecia
In this case cyclophosphamide was responsible for the sudden diffuse hair loss; other cytotoxic drugs, anticoagulants, and an excess of vitamin A may have the same effect.

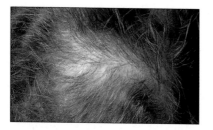

Fig. 4.8 Androgenic alopecia
The hair follicle density is greatly diminished and the involved areas are poorly circumscribed. There is no scarring and on close examination the openings of hair follicles may be seen.

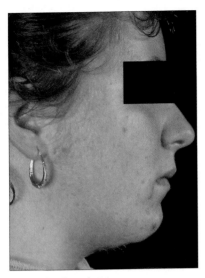

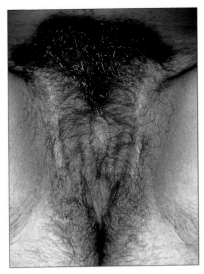

Fig. 4.9 Hirsutism
Look for other evidence of virilization when hirsutism is combined with acne.

Fig. 4.10 Virilization
In this young girl, an adrenal tumour was responsible for severe acne plus hirsutism and clitoromegaly.

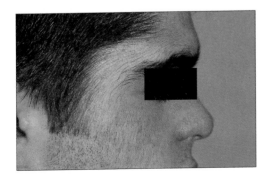

Fig. 4.11 Hypertrichosis
The excessive growth of hair over the temples and on the cheeks is like that seen in porphyria cutanea tarda but no underlying cause was found here.

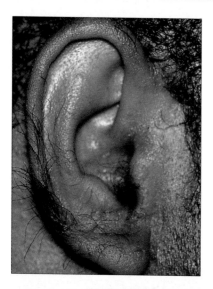

Fig. 4.12 Hairy ears
A curiosity, running in some families and possibly due to a gene on the Y chromosome.

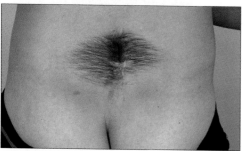

Fig. 4.13 Spina bifida occulta
Hairy patches may provide the clue to the underlying abnormality.

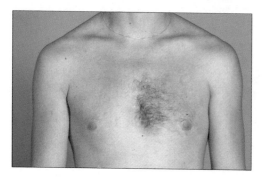

Fig. 4.14 Becker's naevus
These appear at puberty in boys. The naevus is discoloured, shows signs of acne and is more hairy than the rest of the skin. A clonal abnormality of androgen receptors may be responsible.

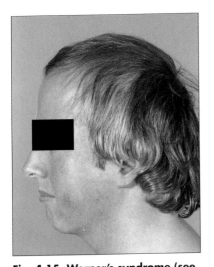

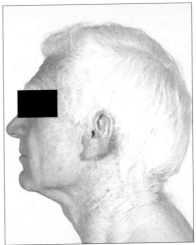

Fig. 4.15 Werner's syndrome (see also Fig. 1.86)

Patient, here aged 26, had already noticed premature greying of the hair for a few years.

Fig. 4.16 Albinism

The presence of freckling around the neck suggests that this patient has tyrosinase-positive (type II) albinism, though the hair is white rather than yellow. The risk of developing squamous cell carcinomas of the skin is high if sun exposure is not avoided.

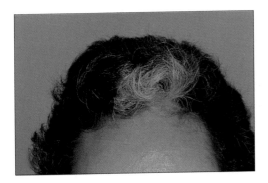

Fig. 4.17 Poliosis

This may be an isolated abnormality (as here) or a part of piebaldism or the Waardenberg syndrome.

THE SCALP

The scalp is a common site for **psoriasis** (Fig. 4.18), **neurodermatitis** and **seborrhoeic eczema**. If the latter is intractible, an underlying HIV infection should be considered.

Bald scalps are exposed to excessive ultraviolet radiation and so are a common site for **actinic keratoses** (Fig. 4.19), **basal cell carcinomas** and **squamous cell carcinomas** (Figs. 1.91 and 1.65–1.67). UV exposure also predisposes to systemic and discoid **lupus erythematosus**, often with alopecia (Fig. 4.1). In **porphyria cutanea tarda**, the scalp may show bullae, erosions and scarring (Fig. 8.19). Other bullous disorders, such as **pemphigoid, pemphigus, epidermolysis bullosa** and **dermatitis herpetiformis** may affect the scalp; a plaque of scarring and blistering there is characteristic of **mucous membrane pemphigoid** (Fig. 4.20).

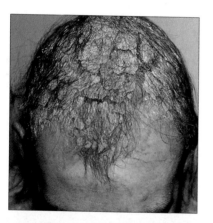

Fig. 4.18 Psoriasis of the scalp
Severe psoriasis can cause a temporary loss of hair when adherent scales are removed but usually psoriasis of the scalp is felt rather than seen.

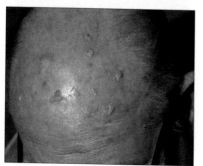

Fig. 4.19 Actinic keratoses
Multiple scalp keratoses, with some pale areas due to previous cryotherapy.

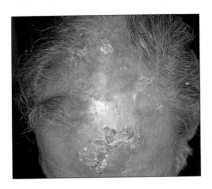

Fig. 4.20 Cicatricial pemphigoid
In this variant (the Brunsting–Perry type)
there are no mucosal lesions. Recurrent
blisters arise on a red plaque, usually, as
here, on the scalp. Scarring leads to
permanent hair loss.

EYES

EYEBROWS

Bushy ones are seen in some **mucopolysaccharidoses** and with drugs such as **diazoxide**. Sparseness is most obvious in the outer third, for example in **hypothyroidism**. Specific dermatoses, such as **alopecia areata** and **follicular mucinosis** (Fig. 4.21), may be limited to the eyebrows.

EYELIDS

The periorbital tissues are lax and oedema readily accumulates there. In atopic eczema an accentuated crease, the **Dennie-Morgan fold**, is common. Ectropion may occur if the skin becomes tight, as in non-bullous **ichthyosiform erythroderma** (Fig. 4.22). The eyelids are a common site for increased pigmentation (Fig. 4.23) which, although usually familial, may be associated with carcinoma of the bronchus or **ochronosis**, in which the sclera is often brown, or follows inflammatory dermatoses. The heliotrope rash of **dermatomyositis** is seen best on the eyelids. Periorbital haemorrhages may be seen in **amyloidosis** (Fig. 4.24) but the most common cause is trauma. **Xanthelasmas** (Fig. 4.25) may be an isolated finding or associated with hyperlipidaemia. They should be distinguished from **syringomas** (Fig. 4.26) which are benign tumours of sweat glands. **Basal cell carcinomas** may approach dangerously near to the eyelids (Fig. 4.27). Scaling and erythema of the eyelids occur in allergic contact dermatitis (Fig. 4.28) and around the eyelashes in seborrhoeic dermatitis which may be an early manifestation of **AIDS**.

In **myxoedema** the lids are puffy (Fig. 7.45); in **hyperthyroidism** there may be lid retraction, chemosis with thick oedematous eyelids and proptosis. In **cicatricial pemphigoid**, adhesions may form between the the upper and lower eyelids (Fig. 4.29).

LACHRYMAL GLANDS

Visibly swollen lachrymal glands may be due to infections, such as **mumps** and **herpes simplex** or to **sarcoidosis**. Tear secretion is often reduced in the elderly and this is also a manifestation of **Sjögren's syndrome**.

FRONT OF THE EYE

In atopic eczema, **keratoconus** may develop — the apex of the cornea bulges progressively to produce a myopic astigmatism. **Conjunctivitis** is a feature of the **Stevens–Johnson syndrome** (Figs. 1.82 and 4.43), **Reiter's disease, Churg-Strauss allergic granulomatosis** and some infections such as **measles** (Fig. 1.9). In **ataxia telangiectasia,** conjunctival telangiectasia may extend onto the eyelids.

If the sclera is thin, as in **osteogenesis imperfecta**, it may look blue as retinal melanin shows through. In **ochronosis**, a black pigment is deposited. **Scleritis** may be associated with connective tissue diseases, such as **rheumatoid arthritis,** or with **polyarteritis nodosa, Wegener's disease, relapsing polychondritis** or **gout**. It also occurs in **herpes zoster** (Figs. 1.96 and 1.111) and **erythema nodosum**.

Acute uveitis is seen in ankylosing spondylitis, inflammatory bowel disease, sarcoidosis, Reiter's disease, viral illness and syphilis. Sarcoidosis causes **chronic uveitis** and Behçet's disease a relapsing one with hypopyon. Flecks of **pigment on the iris** are common and of no significance; translucent irides are seen in oculo-cutaneous albinism, **Lisch nodules**, small melanocytic naevi of the iris (Fig. 4.30), occur in most patients with generalized neurofibromatosis.

BACK OF THE EYE

Angioid streaks (Fig. 4.31) are diagnostic of **pseudo-xanthoma elasticum**. In **tuberous sclerosis**, an astrocytic hamartoma may be seen as a grey patch with an indistinct edge which progresses to a yellowish 'mulberry' tumour. In the **Sturge–Weber syndrome** (Fig. 4.32), a capillary malformation may show up as a small flat lesion in the posterior fundus or as a more diffuse red area looking like velvet; **glaucoma** complicates 30% of cases.

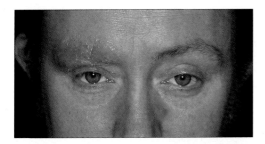

Fig. 4.21 Follicular mucinosis
A favoured site for this condition causing the loss of an eyebrow, it may progress to a cutaneous T cell lymphoma

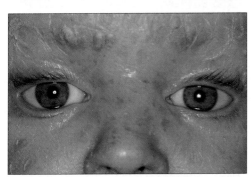

Fig. 4.22 Ectropion
The lower eye lids are everted by the tightness of the skin in this child with ichthyosiform erythroderma.

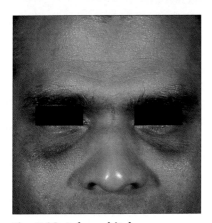

Fig. 4.23 Infra-orbital pigmentation
A common appearance, often, as here, with no detectable cause.

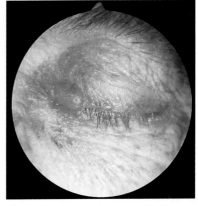

Fig. 4.24 Systemic amyloidosis
Translucent yellowish beading along the margins of the eyelids plus a hint of pinch purpura underneath. The systemic association is with multiple myeloma.

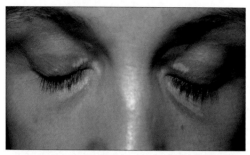

Fig. 4.25 Xanthelasma palpebrarum
As is usually the case these yellowish plaques affect the nasal side of the eyelids. These lesions are common, and often no underlying hyper-lipoproteinaemia can be found.

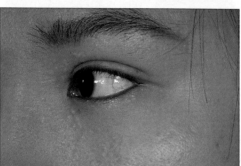

Fig. 4.26 Syringoma
Multiple skin coloured papules — frequently familial.

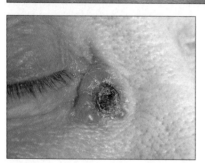

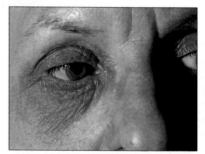

Fig. 4.27 Basal cell carcinoma
Should be removed by an expert to avoid damaging the naso-lacrymal duct. A typical ulcerated nodular basal cell carcinoma. Reproduced with permission from Edwards, Bouchier, Haslett et al (eds), Davidson's Principles and Practice of Medicine, 17th edn., 1995, Churchill-Livingstone, Edinburgh.

Fig. 4.28 Contact dermatitis
The thin skin of the eyelids is a favourite site. This lichenified eczema was an allergic reaction to neomycin in an eyedrop.

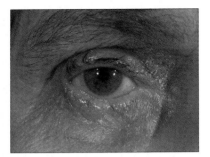

Fig. 4.29 Cicatricial pemphigoid
The other name for this condition, benign mucosal pemphigoid, gives no impression of how severely it can damage the eye. This patient had suffered from conjunctival bullae for many years, and now adhesions have formed between the upper and lower eye lids.

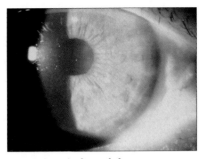

Fig. 4.30 Lisch nodules
Best seen with a slit-lamp — these are small circular pigmented hamartomas of the iris seen in neurofibromatosis.

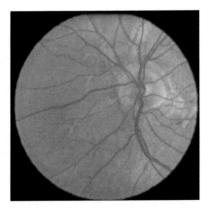

Fig. 4.31 Angioid streaks
Pigmented streaks, broader than the blood vessels with which they are sometimes confused, radiating out from an incomplete grey rim around the optic disc.

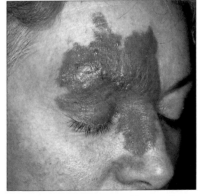

Fig. 4.32 Capillary malformation
Beware of glaucoma when these affect the eyelids.

THE MOUTH

Fordyce spots (Fig. 4.33) are often mistaken for lichen planus (see below) but the small yellowish papules are simply prominent sebaceous glands. About 50% of patients with **lichen planus** (Figs. 4.34 and 4.35) have asymptomatic white lacy lines, dots and occasionally small plaques inside their cheeks. **Oral candidiasis** (Fig. 4.36) causes whitish adherent plaques (like bread sauce) on the mucosa; they wipe off leaving an erythematous base.

Leucoplakia (Fig. 4.37) is not a single condition but a term covering white patches or plaques on the buccal mucosa or tongue which cannot be rubbed off. Lichen planus, Fordyce spots, candidiasis and cheek biting must be excluded. Leucoplakia may be due to smoking or other causes of intra-oral irritation and has a tendency to transform into squamous cell carcinoma. **Hairy leucoplakia** (Fig. 4.38) appears as a corrugated white patch on the side of the tongue. It is seen in severe immunodeficiency, especially with HIV infection and is due to the Epstein–Barr virus. The 'cobble-stone' appearance of the oral mucosa in **Crohn's disease** (Fig. 4.39) should not be confused with leucoplakia.

The commonest mouth ulcers are **aphthous** (Fig. 4.40). They are painful, with a yellowish base and a surrounding red halo. Aphthous ulcers may coincide with iron, folic acid or vitamin B12 deficiency, malabsorption (e.g. in coeliac disease, Crohn's disease) and even the luteal phase of the menstrual cycle. **Behçet's disease** (genital lesions, iritis, arthritis) (Fig. 4.41) should be considered when oral ulcers are unusually large and recurrent. Mouth ulcers are also a sign of **neutropenia**.

A Coxsackie infection causes **hand, foot and mouth disease**, with small aphthous-like ulcers in the mouth and blisters with red halos on the hands and feet. Large buccal blisters or erosions may be the presenting sign of **pemphigus vulgaris** (Fig. 4.42) and are also seen in other bullous diseases such as **dystrophic epidermolyis bullosa**, in which oesophageal involvement may lead to stricture. **Erythema multiforme**, especially its severe form, the **Stevens–Johnson syndrome**, can cause bloody erosions on the lips (Fig. 1.82), buccal mucosa and tongue (Fig. 4.43). The conjunctivae and genitalia (Fig. 1.13) may also be involved.

Buccal pigmentation is normal in blacks. In whites, intra-oral melanosis has to be distinguished from the greyer colour caused by implanted dental amalgam. Buccal pigmentation is also seen in **Addison's disease** (Fig. 4.44) and the **Peutz–Jeghers syndrome** (Figs. 6.7 and 6.8).

A **geographical tongue** (Fig. 4.45) has smooth red areas surrounded by white margins of furred filiform papillae. The patterns change from day to day and the condition is harmless. A large tongue may be a feature of acromegaly (Fig. 4.46). A smooth tongue may also be seen in iron deficiency, pernicious anaemia or malabsorption. A 'raw-beef' tongue, with oral ulceration, is part of the

glucagonoma syndrome (Fig. 4.47). A scrotal tongue, facial nerve palsy and swollen lips make up the Melkersson-Rosenthal syndrome. Primary syphilitic chancres can involve the lips, tongue or palate. Secondary syphilis is characterized by mucous patches and snail-track ulcers. Gummas occasionally involve the palate or tongue.

The gums and teeth also provide clues to general health. **Gingival hyperplasia** may be due to treatment with phenytoin (Fig. 4.48), some calcium channel blockers and cyclosporin. The **teeth** may be present at birth (in pachyonychia congenita), lacking in enamel (dystrophic epidermolysis bullosa), abnormally shaped (congenital syphilis, **ectodermal dysplasias** (Fig. 4.49)) or abnormally coloured (tetracycline treatment in childhood).

Swelling (Fig. 4.50), **telangiectases** (Fig. 4.51), **pigmentation** and **erosions** (Fig. 1.82) of the lips may provide clues to systemic disorders. The lower lip is a common site for **squamous cell carcinoma** (Fig. 4.52). Licking the lips causes chapping (Fig. 4.53).

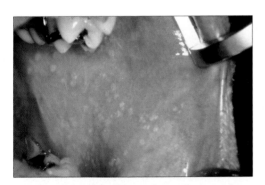

Fig. 4.33 Fordyce spots
These yellowish papules are ectopic sebaceous glands and are common.

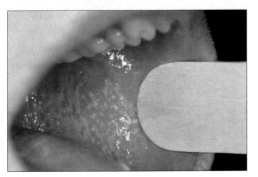

Fig. 4.34 Lichen planus
White dots and a reticulate pattern are both seen in this florid example.

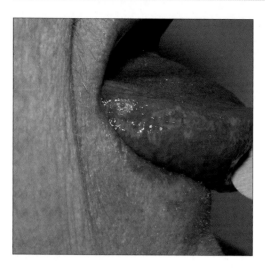

Fig. 4.35 Lichen planus
Delicate reticulate white
tracery is seen along the side
of the tongue in a patient with
widespread lichen planus.

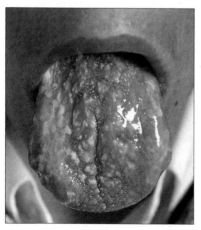

**Fig. 4.36 Chronic mucocutaneous
candidiasis**
This patient also had Addison's disease
and hypoparathyroidism as part of the
candida-endocrinopathy syndrome.

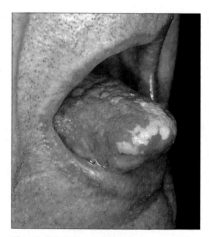

Fig. 4.37 Leucoplakia
These fixed whitish plaques on the
tongue carry a high risk of developing
into a squamous cell carcinoma.
Predisposing factors include smoking,
and occasionally syphilis.

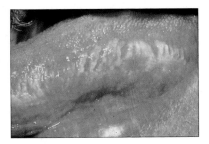

Fig. 4.38 Hairy leucoplakia
Whitish areas on the tongue, here seen in a patient with an HIV infection.

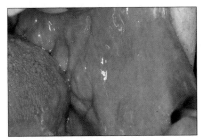

Fig. 4.39 Crohn's disease
An exuberant mucosa with a cobblestone pattern.

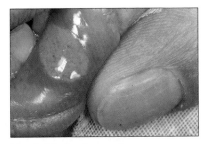

Fig. 4.40 Apthous ulcers
An established but still painful lesion with a typical erythematous halo and a greyish base. This ulcer was on the borderline between minor (2–4mm) and major. In severe cases consider Behçet's syndrome or a deficiency of iron, folic acid or B$_{12}$

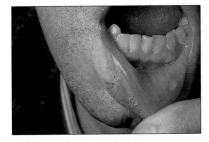

Fig. 4.41 Behçet's syndrome
Painful oral and genital ulcers are an important part of this syndrome, the other features of which include uveiitis, arthralgia, pustulation in response to venepuncture and neurological involvement.

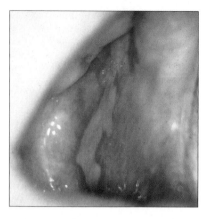

Fig. 4.42 Pemphigus vulgaris
About half of all patients with pemphigus present with lesions in the mouth. This erosion was painful and the condition usually requires treatment with systemic steroids.

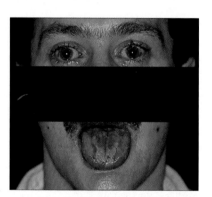

Fig. 4.43 Stevens-Johnson syndrome
Tongue and eye involvement in this drug-induced reaction.

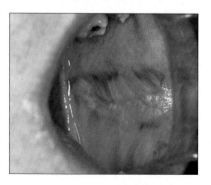

Fig. 4.44 Addison's disease
The same patient as in Figure 4.36 showing obvious pigmentation inside the cheeks as a result of the Addison's disease.

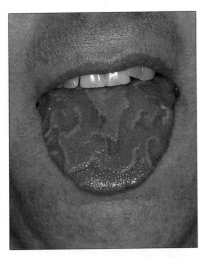

Fig. 4.45 Geographical tongue
The moving pattern of red areas with thickened whitish borders is typical of this common and benign condition. There may be an occasional association with psoriasis and with Reiter's syndrome.

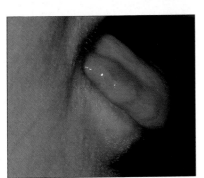

Fig. 4.46 Macroglossia
Pressure from the teeth causes these dents around the edge of the tongue; it may be seen in acromegaly and systemic amyloidosis.

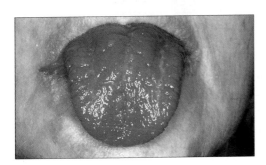

Fig. 4.47 Glucagonoma syndrome
A 'raw-beef' tongue and angular cheilitis. Other features of the syndrome are necrolytic migratory erythema (Fig. 2.3), diabetes, weight loss and diarrhoea. The changes disappeared after removal of the α-cell tumour of the pancreas.

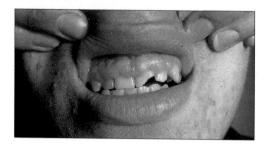

Fig. 4.48 Gingival hyperplasia
Phenytoin therapy leads to fibroblast proliferation. Gingival hyperplasia, as seen here, is one result of this.

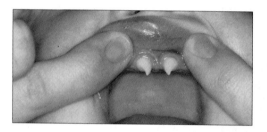

Fig. 4.49 Hypohidrotic ectodermal dysplasis
Conical teeth may be seen in this condition. Other features include diminished sweating, heat intolerance, alopecia and hypoplastic nails.

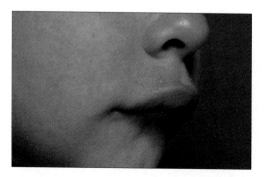

Fig. 4.50 Granulomatous cheilitis
Permanent swelling of the lips may be a feature of Crohn's disease or the Melkersson-Rosenthal syndrome (with a scrotal tongue and recurrent facial nerve paralysis). Rarely it is due to an allergy to constituents of toothpaste. It must be distinguished from evanescent angioedema.

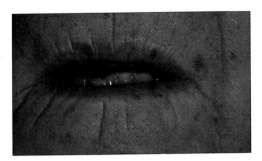

Fig. 4.51 Systemic sclerosis
An increasingly tight mouth which shows radial furrowing plus telangiectasia.

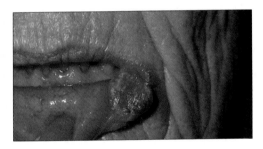

Fig. 4.52 Squamous cell carcinoma
The lower lip is a favourite place; precipitating factors include smoking and excessive exposure to sunlight.

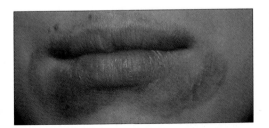

Fig. 4.53 Lip licking
A tiresome habit, difficult to break, usually seen in children with atopic eczema. The dry chapped skin is sore and tends to split; further licking makes it more comfortable in the short term but worse in the end.

NAILS

NAIL STRUCTURE

Normal nails change with age and longitudinal ridging or beading of the nail plate is not significant in the elderly. **Lamellar splitting** (flaking and fragility of the distal end of the nail plate) is commonly seen in housewives.

The coarse pits of **psoriasis** (Fig. 4.54), often accompanied by separation of the nail from the bed (onycholysis (Fig. 4.55)) and by subungual hyperkeratosis are characteristic. Many nails may be affected; in contrast, **fungal infections** tend to involve only a few. Smaller but more irregular pits are seen in eczema and alopecia areata. Crumbling and discolouration of the nails, starting at the free edge and spreading proximally, is likely to be due to a fungal infection (Fig. 4.56). The toe webs should be examined too.

Thinning of the nail plate, with irregular ridges and grooves, occurs in about 10% of patients with **lichen planus**. Less often the cuticle grows forward and over the base of the nail, which it replaces (**pterygium**).

Transverse ridging may follow nail fold eczema or paronychia. Single transverse grooves, lying at the same level in all nails (**Beau's lines**, Fig. 4.57), follow the arrest of nail growth caused by an acute illness. A ladder pattern of transverse ridges, running up the centre of a thumb nail, is usually due to the common habit of **picking at the nail fold** (Fig. 4.58).

Gross thickening and malalignment of the big toe nails (**onychogryphosis** (Fig. 8.29)) follows chronic trauma, from sport or from ill-fitting shoes.

NAIL SHAPE

Clubbing is a bilateral curvature of the nail with enlargement of underlying soft tissues (Fig. 4.59). Loss of the angle between the nail and the nail fold is best seen from the side. The nail bed may be fluctuant. Its causes are numerous and well known. Clubbing must be distinguished from a hook nail which is curved like a claw and most commonly due to trauma.

The spooned nails of **koilonychia** dip in the middle (Fig. 4.60). Initially the nail plate flattens and later full spooning develops. In neonates, koilonychia may be physiological but later in life it is associated with iron deficiency even though the haemoglobin level may remain normal. Koilonychia also occurs in old age, in peripheral arterial disease or after occupational contact with oil.

Long narrow nails (dolichonychia) are seen in Marfan's syndrome, the Ehlers–Danlos syndrome, hypopituitarism and in eunuchs.

Short nails (brachyonychia), wider than they are long, are often due to nail biting but may occur after resorption of the terminal phalanx in hyperparathyroidism or psoriatic arthropathy. **Nail en racquette** is most obvious on the thumbs and may be familial.

Sometimes nails are partly or completely absent, either as an isolated defect, or after lichen planus, the Stevens–Johnson syndrome, chronic graft versus host disease or amyloidosis.

ABNORMAL NAIL COLOUR

Nails contain melanin and their degree of pigmentation is a **racial characteristic** — the darker the skin, the more pigmented the nails. **Multiple dark streaks** are common in Afro-Caribbeans but unusual in Caucasians in whom they may be a clue to Addison's disease. **A single dark streak** raises the possibility of a melanocytic naevus (Fig. 4.61), or even a melanoma, arising in the nail matrix.

Without a history of trauma, a **subungual haemorrhage** may be hard to tell from a **melanoma**. The former will grow out (Fig. 4.62) and in the latter, the nearby skin becomes pigmented too (**Hutchinson's sign**) (Fig. 4.63). Smaller haemorrhages take up a '**splinter**' shape (Fig. 4.64) following the longitudinal ridging of the nail bed. Most splinter haemorrhages are due to trauma rather than subacute bacterial endocarditis.

Infections can also discolour the nails. Overgrowth of **pseudomonas**, often in an area of onycholysis, gives a striking green colour (Fig. 4.65). The adjacent nail plate can turn a dirty brown or grey in chronic **monilial or bacterial paronychia**, and a chalky yellow colour in chronic **Scopulariopsis** infections. The white colour of **dermatophyte infections** of the nail plate is most obvious in the superficial type (Fig. 4.66).

Punctate, linear or total **leuconychia** may be traumatic or inherited (Figs. 4.67 and 4.68). However, an unusual whiteness, extending up to within 2-3mm of the free margin, can be seen in some cases of cirrhosis (**Terry's nail**). The '**half and half**' **nails** of chronic renal failure have a proximal whitish and distal reddish-brown part (Fig. 4.69).

Some **drugs** discolour the nails: examples include minocycline, zidovudine, and chloroquine. Tetracyclines and psoralens are the most common causes of photo-onycholysis. **Blue lunules** are seen in argyria (Fig. 4.70); azure ones in Wilson's disease; and pink ones in congestive heart failure.

The discoloured nails of the **yellow nail syndrome** are thick, hard, and over-curved from side to side (Fig. 4.71). They grow very slowly. The internal components of the syndrome are lymphoedema, pleural effusions and chronic respiratory disorders such as bronchiectasis.

Nails may also pick up colour from their environment, for example during smoking (Fig. 4.72) or after contact with hair dyes or potassium permanganate. When growing out, the proximal edge of the exogenous pigment retains the shape of the nail fold.

NAIL FOLDS

An intact cuticle protects the nail fold from infection. **Acute paronychia** may follow cuticular damage and is usually of only one finger. In contrast, **chronic paronychia** (Fig. 4.73) occurs in those whose hands are often in water, or in patients with diabetes, Raynaud's phenomenon or skin diseases such as eczema or psoriasis. Herpetic whitlows are very painful.

The periungual tissues are also inflamed in **acrodermatitis enteropathica** which occurs in zinc deficient children. The main eruption lies around the mouth and nose and in the anogenital region. Hair loss is an important feature.

Ragged cuticles may be due to trauma but are also seen in **dermatomyositis**. An associated erythema often runs along the extensor tendons (**Dowling's Lines**) (Fig. 2.41) and smooth, purplish papules (**Gottron's papules**) lie on the backs of the knuckles (Fig. 5.18). **Nail fold telangiectasia** (Fig. 4.74) is a good indicator of the presence of a collagen vascular disease. Papules on the nail folds may be **viral warts** (Fig. 4.75), naevi, or fibromas. In **tuberous sclerosis**, periungual fibromas (Fig. 4.76) appear in adult life and should trigger a search for other features such as ash leaf macules, adenoma sebaceum (Figs. 1.59 and 5.29), connective tissue naevi (Fig. 7.15) and retinal phacomata.

Myxoid cysts, containing a thick, clear fluid, affect the proximal nail fold and may cause a linear depression of the adjacent nail plate (Figs. 1.131 and 4.77).

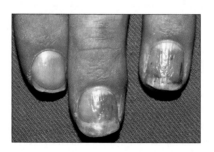

Fig. 4.54 Psoriasis of the nail
Pitting and distal separation of the nail plate from the nailbed (onycholysis).

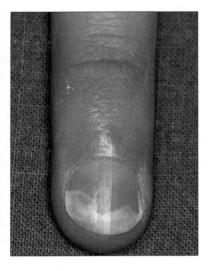

Fig. 4.55 Onycholysis
Separation of the nail plate from the nail bed is common. Medical causes are said to include thyrotoxicosis. Here the surface pitting on the nails suggests that the condition was due to psoriasis.

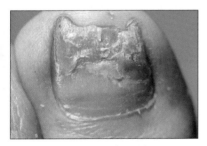

Fig. 4.56 Fungal infections
The distal half of the big toe nail has become thickened, discoloured and crumbly.

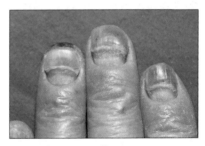

Fig. 4.57 Beau's lines
A very gross example caused by a severe drug reaction. The distal parts of the nails will soon be shed.

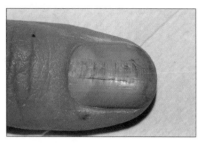

Fig. 4.58 Habit tic nail dystrophy
Picking or rubbing at the cuticle creates a ladder pattern of transverse ridges and furrows running up the centre of one or both thumb nails.

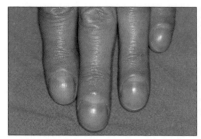

Fig. 4.59 Clubbing
Clubbing here was familial rather than an indicator of any underlying abnormality.

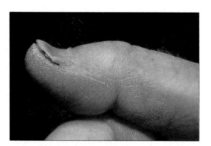

Fig. 4.60 Koilonychia
If all the nails are spoon-shaped, as here, think of iron deficiency.

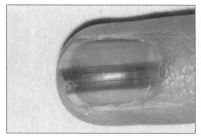

Fig. 4.61 Melanocytic naevus
Longitudinal pigmented streaks are normal in some races. However, this broad dark band was due to a junctional melanocytic naevus in the nail matrix.

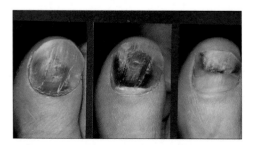

Fig. 4.62 Subungual haematoma
These three pictures show a subungual haematoma growing out over the course of six months. The patient was unaware of having damaged the area, and the differential diagnosis when he was first seen had to include a malignant melanoma.

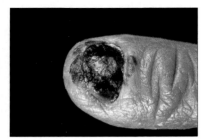

Fig. 4.63 Malignant melanoma
An important feature here is the spread to involve the proximal nail fold (Hutchinson's sign).

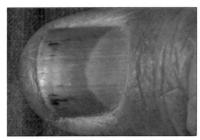

Fig. 4.64 Splinter haemorrhages
The characteristic linear shape of these lesions is determined by the longitudinal ridges and grooves in the nail bed. Most, particularly the distal ones, are due to minor trauma. Proximal splinters may be a part of subacute bacterial endocarditis.

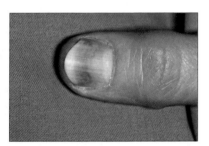

Fig. 4.65 Onycholysis
The green colour is due to the overgrowth of pseudomonas aeruginosa where the nail plate has separated from its bed.

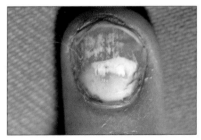

Fig. 4.66 Nail tinea
A superficial white type of onychomycosis, here due to trichophyton rubrum.

Fig. 4.67 Leuconychia
This punctate type of leuconychia signifies nothing more than minor trauma.

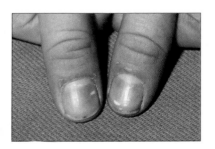

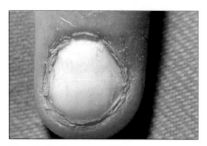

Fig. 4.68 Leuconychia
The whiteness of this patient's nails had been present since birth; an acquired whiteness hints at hypoalbuminaemia.

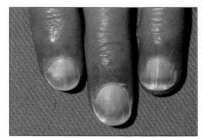

Fig. 4.69 'Half and half' nail
This slide shows three features. The 'half and half' nails signify renal failure — the proximal nail is white and distal one third is pink. Telangiectasia of the proximal nail fold is due to systemic lupus erythematosus. The wart may be a sign of immunodeficiency.

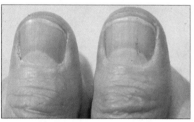

Fig. 4.70 Argyria
The cause here was an excessive use of silver-containing throat antiseptic. The nails have a typical bluish colour.

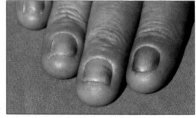

Fig. 4.71 Yellow nail syndrome
Apart from their yellowish colour, these nails are abnormal in that they grow very slowly and are slightly thickened. Lymphoedema is an important part of the syndrome. Lymphatic abnormalities may lead to recurrent pleural effusions. Other associated conditions include bronchiectasis, the nephrotic syndrome and AIDS.

Fig. 4.72 Cigarette smoking
Nails heavily stained with tar are often seen in patients with carcinoma of the lung.

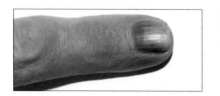

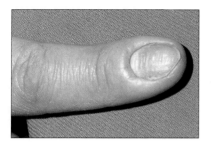

Fig. 4.73 Chronic paronychia
The ridging and discolouration of the nail plate is secondary to recurrent bouts of inflammation of the proximal nail fold. The cuticle is lost. This condition is seen particularly in diabetics and those with a poor peripheral circulation.

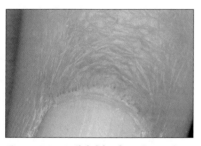

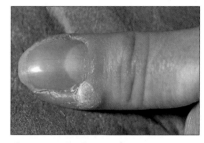

Fig. 4.74 Nail fold telangiectasia
This striking example was seen in a patient with the CRST variant of systemic sclerosis.

Fig. 4.75 Periungual wart
A typical example.

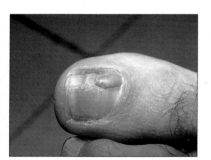

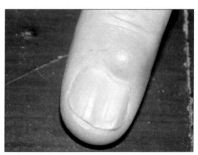

Fig. 4.76 Periungual fibroma
These are seen in adults with tuberous sclerosis.

Fig. 4.77 Myxoid cyst
These benign cysts discharge their mucoid contents in response to minor trauma but usually refill. A longitudinal groove is often seen in the nail plate adjacent to the cyst.

GENITAL AND PERIANAL

The skin in these areas is warm, moist and subject to maceration and fissuring. This is made worse by obesity, sweating, urinary and faecal incontinence and by friction. **Intertrigo** is therefore common in infants and the elderly (Fig. 3.4). Many dermatoses here have infective causes, such as **Candida albicans, dermatophyte fungi** (Fig. 4.78) or **staphylococci**, or are due to localized **eczema** or **psoriasis**. If intertigo is intractible, **diabetes mellitus** must be considered. Perianal bacterial infections are common in leukaemic and other **immunosuppressed patients**.

Pruritus may lead to secondary lichenification of the genital or perianal skin. Often no cause can be found but it is important to consider atopic and contact dermatitis, psoriasis, diabetes mellitus and pubic lice, scabies (Fig. 4.79), or the rare extramammary Paget's disease (Fig. 4.80). **Vulval itch** may be due to **lichen sclerosus et atrophicus** involving the vulval and perianal areas. The features are distinctive (Fig. 4.81). The most important complication is squamous cell carcinoma (Fig. 4.82). In men, lichen sclerosus may cause phimosis (Fig. 4.83). Perianal lesions are common in **Crohn's disease** (Fig. 4.84) and include oedematous tags, perianal maceration, inflammatory swellings, fistulae and ischiorectal abscesses.

The small painful vesicles of **herpes genitalis** break down to erosions which heal in about 10 days. **Anogenital zoster** is less common but may be a presenting feature of AIDS. **Behçet's disease** may present with genital ulceration (Fig. 4.85). **Condylomata accuminata** (viral warts) (Fig. 4.86) can usually be distinguished from syphilitic condylomata lata which are flat.

Perineal pigmentation increases in pregnancy and in Addison's disease. Acanthosis nigricans usually affects the groins and internal malignancy and diabetes mellitus should always be considered as a possible underlying cause.

Candidiasis is the most common cause of **balanitis** but a persistent circinate balanitis may accompany Reiter's syndrome (Fig. 4.87). In situ malignancy of the glans appears as an enlarging shiny velvety plaque (Fig. 4.88); biopsy is indicated. The genitalia are often involved in **fixed drug eruptions** (Fig. 4.89).

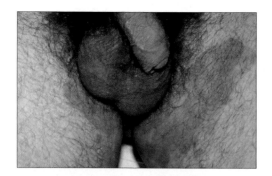

Fig. 4.78 Tinea cruris
An extensive infection with
trichophyton rubrum which
responded well to terbinafine
therapy.

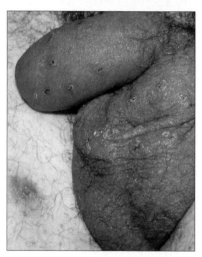

**Fig. 4.79 Scabies of the penis and
scrotum**
These excoriated scrotal nodules can only
be due to scabies: look for further
evidence elsewhere.

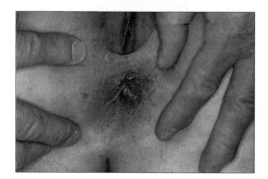

**Fig. 4.80
Extramammary Paget's
disease**
Paget's disease can occur
away from the nipple, and is
shown here as a red velvet
plaque at the anal orifice. It
provided the first clue to a
carcinoma of the rectum (see
also Fig. 1.77).

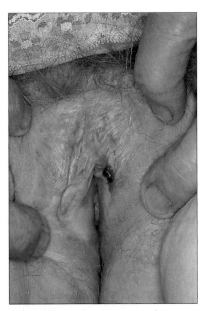

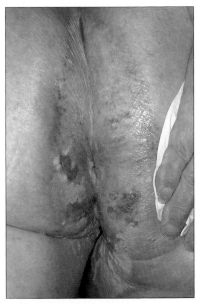

Fig. 4.81 Lichen sclerosus et atrophicus
The vulva is a common site for this condition which can be the precursor of squamous cell carcinoma.

Fig. 4.82 Lichen sclerosus et atrophicus
Biopsy confirmed that the lesion seen beside the anus was an early squamous cell carcinoma.

Fig. 4.83 Lichen sclerosus et atrophicus
The whitish discolouration of the foreskin is typical of this condition which can cause phimosis and hence urinary obstruction.

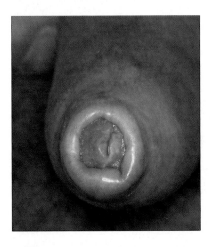

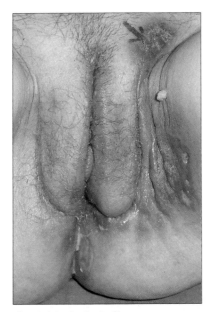

Fig. 4.84 Crohn's disease
Multiple granulomatous lesions, tags and
sinuses are seen here in the groin folds.

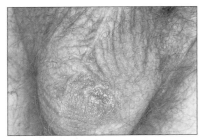

Fig. 4.85 Behçet's syndrome
Persistent genital ulcers are an important
part of this condition.

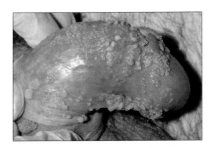

**Fig. 4.86 Penile warts
(condylomata accuminata)**
A gross example — check for other
sexually transmissible diseases.

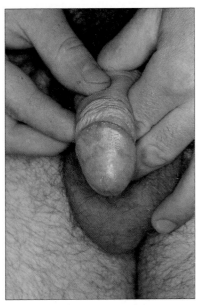

Fig. 4.87 Circinate balanitis
This is often a feature of Reiter's
syndrome.

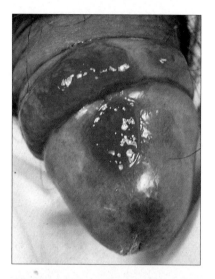

Fig. 4.88 Erythroplasia of Queyrat
Characteristic shiny red areas. These are
often the precursor to a squamous cell
carcinoma of the penis.

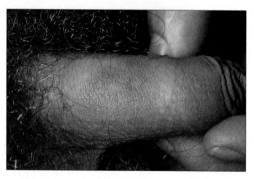

**Fig. 4.89 Fixed drug
eruption**
The penis is a common site.
Tetracycline was responsible
for this lesion, here shown in
the inactive stage of post-
inflammatory
hyperpigmentation. A further
tablet would cause the area to
become red, swollen and
perhaps vesicular.

Chapter 5

Mimicry

Overall impressions are useful. Sometimes, even if the primary lesions have proved hard to identify, it may still be worthwhile recognizing that an eruption looks like one of the commoner dermatoses.

PSORIASIFORM

The plaques of **psoriasis** are well defined, erythematous and covered with silvery scales. They may take up several patterns (large plaque, small plaque, guttate, flexural etc.) and their appearance varies with their site (e.g. flexural lesions may not be scaly (Fig.3.6)). Nevertheless, the diagnosis is usually easy (Figs. 5.1 and 5.2) although pustular varieties of psoriasis may be confusing (Figs. 1.117–1.119 and 5.3).

Several **internal disorders** occur especially in psoriatics. Arthropathy (Fig. 5.4) affects some 5%, involvement of the terminal interphalangeal joints being particularly common (Fig. 5.5). Alcoholism, pemphigoid (Fig. 1.106), Crohn's disease and ulcerative colitis are also associated with psoriasis more often than by chance. Psoriasis may worsen, or appear for the first time in those infected with HIV. Psoriasis may also be made worse by several drugs including **lithium** and **antimalarials**. **Beta-blockers** can both exacerbate psoriasis and themselves cause a psoriasiform drug eruption (Fig. 5.6).

Other conditions to bear in mind include **Reiter's syndrome** (Fig. 5.7), **pityriasis rubra pilaris** (Fig. 5.8), **Bowen's disease** (Fig. 5.47), **Paget's disease** (Fig. 1.76), **discoid lupus erythematosus** (Fig. 1.23), **discoid eczema, acrodermatitis enteropathica** and **inflammatory linear verrucose naevus** (Fig. 2.37).

The term '**parapsoriasis**' has caused confusion for many years. It refers to lesions which look like psoriasis in some ways (redness and scaling) but which differ in more important ways (histology, fixity, failure to respond to treatment). A '**benign**' type of parapsoriasis (Fig. 5.9) contrasts with a '**premycotic**' type which may turn into a cutaneous T cell lymphoma (**mycosis fungoides**) (Figs. 5.10, 5.11 and 1.75).

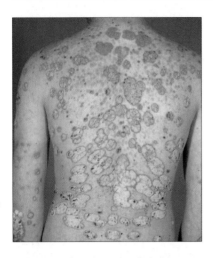

Fig. 5.1 Psoriasis
A severe example, with many thick plaques scattered widely over the trunk and limbs.

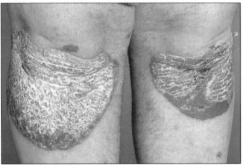

Fig. 5.2 Psoriasis
Psoriasis is commonly seen on the points of the knees. The stubborn variety shown here was unusual in the degree of hyperkeratosis which obstructed topical treatment.

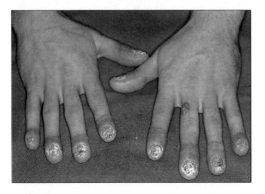

Fig. 5.3 Acrodermatitis continua
A marginated psoriasiform redness is seen on the tips of the digits. There are severe associated nail changes. Pustules can be seen from time to time around the nails. This condition is probably a type of chronic pustular psoriasis.

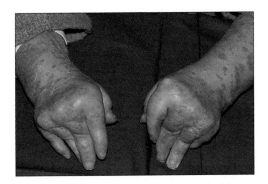

Fig. 5.4 Arthritis mutilans
Inflamed psoriasis on the forearms and hands. The fingers are shortened, floppy and useless for gripping.

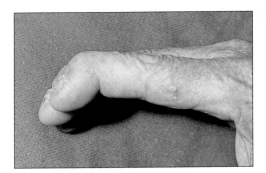

Fig. 5.5 Psoriatic arthropathy
A severe and fixed deformity of the terminal interphalangeal joints. Minor psoriasis of the fingers and marked nail dystrophy can also be seen.

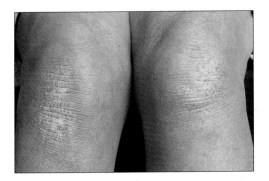

Fig. 5.6 Psoriasiform drug eruption
This hyperkeratosis of the knees shows some resemblance to psoriasis but is too powdery. It was a reaction to beta-blocker medication.

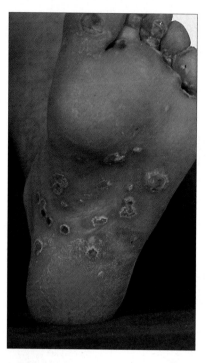

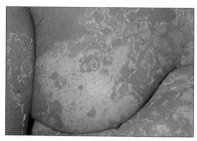

Fig. 5.7 Keratoderma blenorrhagicum
This is one of the skin lesions of Reiter's disease. Thickened limpet-like psoriasiform lesions on the soles are typical.

Fig. 5.8 Pityriasis rubra pilaris
Here obvious follicular involvement can be seen as well as the more extensive red psoriasiform areas. The scaling is too marginate for psoriasis.

Fig. 5.9 Parapsoriasis
This type of parapsoriasis is benign in the sense that it does not evolve into mycosis fungoides. The finger-like processes, stretching around the flanks, are typical, as is their yellowish-red colour.

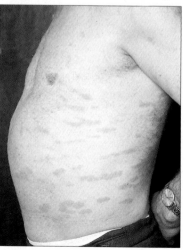

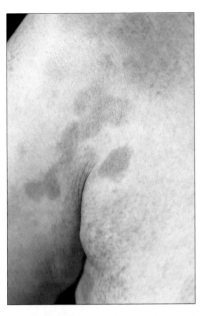

Fig. 5.10 Parapsoriasis
These fixed erythematous areas have less obvious scaling than benign parapsoriasis. The mixture of pigmentation and skin atrophy seen in some areas suggests this may be a prelude to a T cell lymphoma.

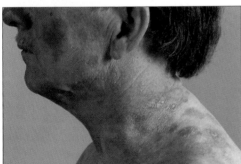

Fig. 5.11 Cutaneous T cell lymphoma
Fixed and irregular psoriasiform plaques had been present for years. The enlarged cervical node had appeared recently. (See also Fig. 1.75.)

LICHENOID

This means looking like **lichen planus** — in which violaceous, intensely itchy, flat-topped papules are found, most often on the extremities and particularly on the volar aspects of the wrists (Fig. 5.12–5.15). White asymptomatic streaking is also found inside the cheeks in about 50% of patients with cutaneous lichen planus (Figs. 4.34 and 4.35). Similar streaking may be a reaction to old amalgam fillings.

Eruptions looking very like lichen planus can be caused by **a variety of drugs** including gold, antimalarials, thiazide diuretics, streptomycin, isoniazid, beta-blockers (Fig. 5.16) and non-steroidal anti-inflammatory drugs. A lichenoid eruption may also be part of chronic **graft versus host disease**.

Other conditions resembling lichen planus include **plane warts** (Fig. 5.17), when a Koebner reaction may add to the confusion, **lichenification** secondary to scratching, **Gottron's papules** (Fig. 5.18) and conditions in which papular deposits appear in the skin, such as **lichen amyloidosus** (Fig. 5.19) and **myxoedematosus** (Fig. 1.46).

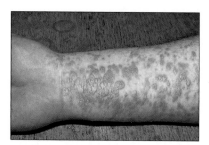

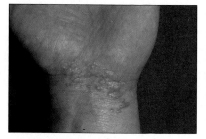

Fig. 5.12 Lichen planus
The typical violaceous colour of the flat-topped and shiny papules of lichen planus is well shown here.

Fig. 5.13 Lichen planus
A group of papules in a favourite area on the flexor aspect of the wrist. Some of the larger lesions show whitish streaks (Wickham's striae).

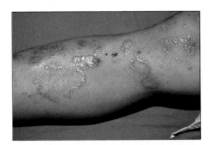

Fig. 5.14 Lichen planus
A view of the leg illustrating the shininess of lichen planus and its tendency to form rings.

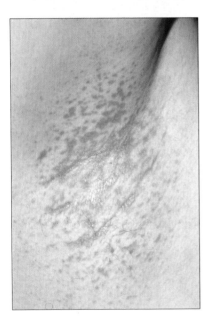

Fig. 5.15 Lichen planus
Lichen planus, as it fades, flattens and leaves macular areas of hyperpigmentation.

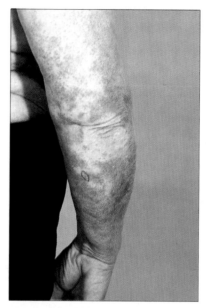

Fig. 5.16 A lichenoid drug eruption
Here due to a beta blocker.

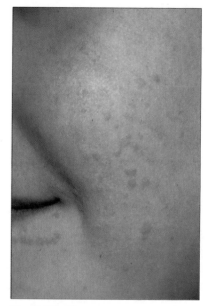

Fig. 5.17 Plane warts
Common, inconspicuous and often hard to treat. The fawn colour is typical as is the line of warts along the scratch mark under the lip (Koebner phenomenon).

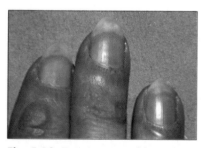

Fig. 5.18 Dermatomyositis
The dilated nail fold capillaries and ragged cuticles are well shown in this close-up view, as are the shiny papules on the backs of the fingers (Gottron's papules).

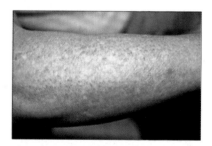

Fig. 5.19 Lichen amyloidosus
This forearm shows large numbers of tiny papules, due to infiltration with amyloid material. This purely local type of amyloidosus is usually itchy and may even be a response to vigorous rubbing.

ACNEIFORM

Ordinary acne is confined to the face and upper trunk (Fig. 5.20 and 5.21). The skin there tends to be greasy and individual lesions include comedones, open and closed, inflamed papules, pustules, nodules and cysts. If the distribution is unusual, or if comedones predominate, an **exogenous cause**, perhaps occupational, should be suspected (Fig. 5.22). Possible culprits include oils or oily cosmetics, tars (Fig. 5.23) and chlorinated hydrocarbons. Sometimes an acneiform eruption occurs as a response to local pressure (e.g. in '**fiddler's neck**') (Fig. 5.24). 'Senile' comedones are common and of little importance. Acneiform lesions in prepubertal children (Fig. 5.25) should prompt an examination for other signs of virilization unless they are naevoid (Fig. 5.26).

A **fulminating acne** (Fig. 5.27) may be associated with fever, leukocytosis and polyarthralgia. Acne may also be one component of **virilization**, and of **Apert's syndrome, suppurative hidradenitis** (Fig. 1.137), **dissecting cellulitis** of the scalp and **steatocystoma multiplex** (Fig. 1.130). Acneiform eruptions may also be due to a variety of drugs including corticosteroids (Fig. 5.28), androgens, lithium, oral contraceptives, iodides, bromides, anti-tuberculosis drugs and anticonvulsants.

An early **adenoma sebaceum** (Fig. 5.29) is occasionally mistaken for acne; a more common confusion is with **rosacea**, which can be complicated by rhinophyma, lymphoedema and keratitis (Fig. 1.26). Rosacea itself may be confused with the erythema and puffiness caused by dermatomyositis, polycythaemia and, rarely, superior vena caval obstruction.

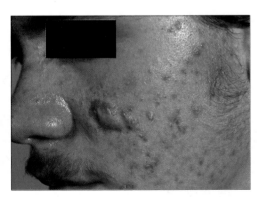

Fig. 5.20 Acne vulgaris
Typical severe acne showing a greasy skin, comedones and inflamed papules and cystic lesions on the cheek.

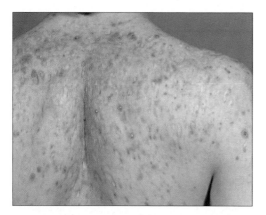

Fig. 5.21 Acne vulgaris
A typical example of severe
acne of the back showing
active pustules and
erythematous papules together
with extensive scarring.

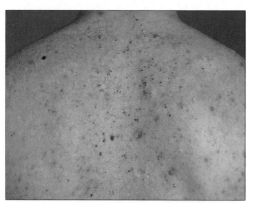

**Fig. 5.22 Exogenous
acne**
The presence of many
comedones, shown here on
the back, should make one
suspect an occupational
cause, such as contact with tar
or chlorinated hydrocarbons.

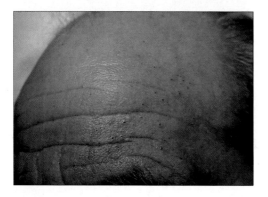

**Fig. 5.23 Exogenous
acne**
This pitch worker showed the
combination of numerous
comedones on exposed areas
plus increasing pigmentation
of the skin.

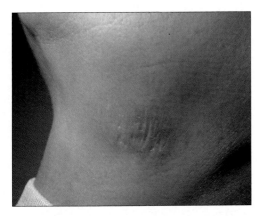

Fig. 5.24 Fiddler's neck
This is a mechanically induced acneiform area due to pressure from a violin.

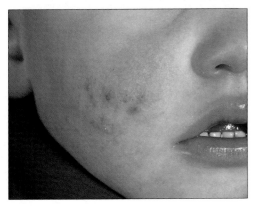

Fig. 5.25 Prepubertal acne
Acne on the face of a young child. This is occasionally a reaction to an androgen-secreting tumour. In infants it may be due to transfer of adrenal androgens in utero.

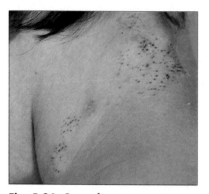

Fig. 5.26 Comedone naevus
These isolated groups of comedones have
been present since birth.

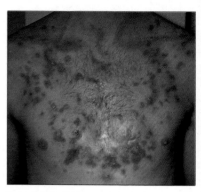

Fig. 5.27 Severe acne
An explosive onset of haemorrhagic acne
may coexist with arthralgia and fever.

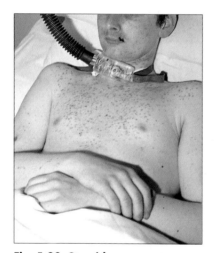

Fig. 5.28 Steroid acne
Some drugs can induce acne. They
include isoniazid, some anti-epileptic
drugs, lithium, iodides and bromides. This
patient developed a monomorphic crop of
small acne spots while taking systemic
corticosteroids.

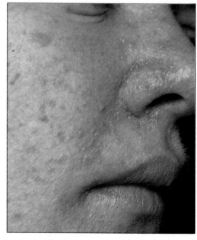

Fig. 5.29 Adenoma sebaceum
Another condition which can in its early
stages look a little like acne. The greasy
skin made this an easy mistake to make
here. In fact it is a part of tuberous
sclerosis.

URTICARIAL

Many conditions can look like urticaria (Figs. 1.32 and 5.30). So-called '**papular urticaria**' is nothing more than an excessive, possibly allergic, reaction to insect bites and stings (Fig. 2.26). **Urticarial vasculitis** (Fig. 5.31) leaves bruising in its wake and its individual lesions last longer than 24 hours. The **figurate erythemas** (Figs. 2.1–2.6) are more fixed and last longer than urticaria (Fig. 1.32). Some **bullous disorders** (e.g. dermatitis herpetiformis and pemphigoid) feature urticarial areas as well as their diagnostic blisters. Sometimes **erythema multiforme** and **annular erythema** have a marked urticarial element. **Sweet's disease** (Fig. 5.32), **fixed drug eruptions** (Fig. 5.33), **erysipelas** (Fig. 1.4) and **dermatomyositis** (Fig. 5.34) may resemble urticaria or angioedema.

Finally, the term **urticaria pigmentosa** describes the various conditions in which the skin contains an excess of mast cells (Figs. 5.35–5.37). All share a tendency to wheal after the skin has been rubbed (Fig. 5.38). Their importance relates to the rare occasions when they are associated with systemic mastocytosis. Such patients may flush repeatedly and are at risk of developing histamine shock. Internal organs involved include the bone marrow, liver and spleen. The **inherited type of angioedema** has been dealt with earlier (Fig. 1.35). **Granulomatous cheilitis** (Fig. 4.50) can simulate angioedema.

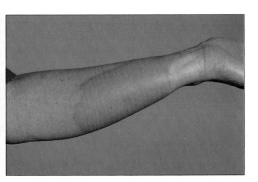

Fig. 5.30 Reaction to a wasp sting
A dramatic, presumably allergic, urticaria-like reaction occurred each time this patient was stung by a wasp.

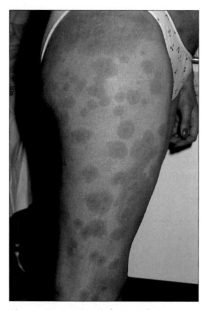

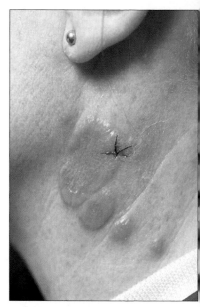

Fig. 5.31 Urticarial vasculitis
The slightly bruised appearance of the centre of these extensive urticarial lesions suggests an underlying vasculitis. The condition may be associated with arthralgia, and occasionally with renal involvement.

Fig. 5.32 Sweet's syndrome
These oedematous plaques are heavily infiltrated with mature polymorphs. The condition may be associated with a high fever, a raised ESR and a high neutrophil count. The most important internal association is with acute myeloid leukaemia.

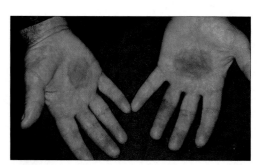

Fig. 5.33 Fixed drug eruption
These areas became swollen and urticarial only when the patient took sulphonamides internally. Later the areas flattened and became pigmented.

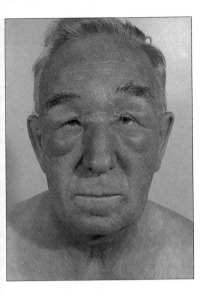

Fig. 5.34 Dermatomyositis
The gross swelling of this patient's face looked almost like angioedema but was in fact due to dermatomyositis.

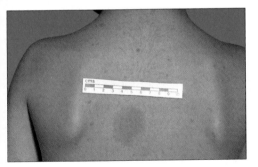

Fig. 5.35 Urticaria pigmentosa
This wheal and flare followed friction to one of the small accumulations of mast cells in this patient with urticaria pigmentosa.

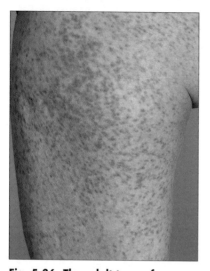

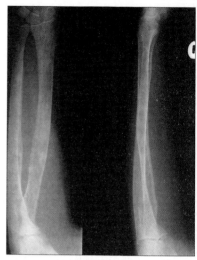

Fig. 5.36 The adult type of mastocytosis
Some of the lesions are telangiectatic. Bone marrow involvement occurs but is uncommon.

Fig. 5.37 Mastocytosis
This patient had extensive cutaneous mastocytosis as well as rarefaction of the bones due to internal involvement, eventually causing a stress fracture of the wrist.

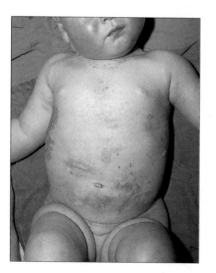

Fig. 5.38 Mastocytosis — diffuse type
This child had diffuse cutaneous mastocytosis. Persistent dermographic wheals appeared after minor friction. Recurrent flushing due to histamine release was also a problem. The condition improved with age, even though mast cell infiltration led to hepatosplenomegaly.

WARTY

Viral warts (Figs. 5.39–5.41) present few diagnostic problems. Those on the hands are usually skin-coloured with a rough surface or protruding finger-like projections (Fig. 5.39). Black, pin-point dots (thrombosed capillaries) may be seen on the surface and are more obvious after paring. Pressure flattens warts on the soles and heels but otherwise they either look like hand warts or adopt a mosaic pattern (Fig. 5.40). The presence of viral warts seldom points to internal problems, but an unusually profuse crop may reflect immunosuppression (either acquired or iatrogenic) (Fig. 5.41), or be due to **epidermodysplasia verruciformis**. This rare condition is characterized by extensive plane warts due to unusual types of human papillomavirus. The skin lesions may become carcinomatous. Cutaneous horns (Fig. 5.42) are warty and affect the elderly.

Skin coloured papules resembling plane warts (**acrokeratosis verruciformis**) on the backs of both hands, are seen in **Darier's disease**. Follicular hyperkeratoses elsewhere (Fig. 5.43), palmar pits (Fig. 5.44) and distinctive nail changes, confirm the diagnosis.

Seborrhoeic warts (Figs. 5.45 and 5.46), often multiple, are common in middle and old age. They usually have a distinctive 'stuck on' appearance but may be flat or pedunculated. Their colour ranges from gingery-yellow to dark brown and their surface shows greasy scaling and scattered keratin plugs. Warty Bowen's disease (Fig. 5.47) may look similar. A sudden eruption of itchy and profuse seborrhoeic warts may signal an underlying carcinoma (**sign of Leser Trélat**) or be the first sign of **acanthosis nigricans** (Figs. 5.48–5.50). Some Afro-Caribbeans have, on their faces, many small dark warty papules which histologically are like seborrhoeic warts (**dermatosis papulosa nigra**) (Fig. 5.51).

Skin tags (acrochordon) (Fig. 5.52) are also common in those over 40. They are most common in the obese and less so in tuberous sclerosis (Figs. 5.29 and 1.59), acanthosis nigricans (Figs. 5.48–5.50), neurofibromatosis (Fig. 3.23), acromegaly and late-onset diabetes. The lesions of molluscum contagiosum, caused by a pox virus, should not be mistaken for tags (Fig. 5.53).

Punctate keratoses of the palms (Fig. 5.54) are now seldom due to arsenic (Fig. 5.55) (an ingredient in so many medicines in the thirties) and are usually an inherited trait.

Some **epidermal naevi** are warty (Figs. 5.56 and 5.57). Extensive ones adopt a bizarre pattern of lines and whorls ('Blaschko's lines'). These stem from the developmental migration of a clone of mutated cells. Extensive epidermal naevi may be associated with defects in other tissues, especially the central nervous system and skeleton (Fig. 2.34).

Blistering in the rare sex-linked dominant condition of **incontinentia pigmenti** (Fig. 10.5) is followed by a warty phase, which in turn is replaced by whorled pigmentation. Associated abnormalities are common and include defects of the central nervous system, eyes, teeth and skeleton.

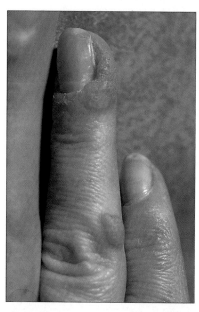

Fig. 5.39 Viral Warts
Viral warts are easy to diagnose but may be difficult to treat. These stubborn examples on a finger eventually cleared only after repeated cryotherapy.

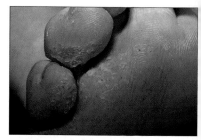

Fig. 5.40 Mosaic warts
Paring shows that these are made up of myriads of tiny warts packed together into a mosaic pattern. Painless but hard to treat.

Fig. 5.41 Viral Warts
A careful look at the individual lesions positioned around the hyperkeratotic plaques shows that they are viral warts. The patient had sarcoidosis; and an associated immunodeficiency allowed the warts to proliferate to this extraordinary extent.

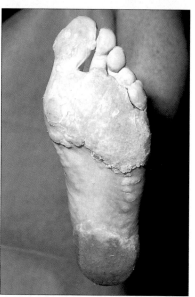

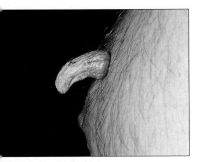

Fig. 5.42 Cutaneous horn

These are common in elderly people, usually on exposed areas. This longstanding keratotic protrusion was easily removed by curettage. Histological examination is essential as a minority of horns arise on an early squamous cell carcinoma.

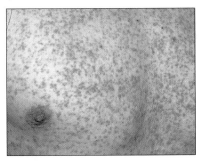

Fig. 5.43 Darier's disease (keratosis follicularis)

Sunburn triggered this eruption of greasy, yellow-brown warty papules on the upper trunk. Later they became luxuriant and odorous after colonization with Gram-negative organisms. Darier's disease is inherited as an autosomal dominant trait.

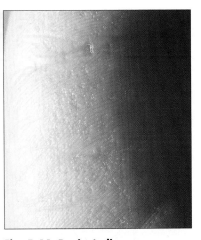

Fig. 5.44 Darier's disease (keratosis follicularis)

Pits on the palms and palmar aspects of the fingers are characteristic of Darier's disease.

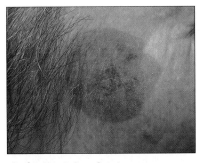

Fig. 5.45 Seborrhoeic wart

This lesion shows much variation in its pigmentation, and the possibility of a lentigo maligna was raised. However, the absence of an irregular edge, and the obvious wartiness seen centrally, suggested that it was a flat seborrhoeic keratosis. Biopsy confirmed this.

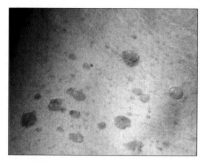

Fig. 5.46 Multiple seborrhoeic warts

These are common, benign, often multiple, and without internal associations apart, perhaps, from the so-called 'sign of Leser-Trélat' in which a sudden eruption of itchy seborrhoeic keratoses is reputed to signal the presence of an underlying neoplasm. It if exists at all, this association is rare.

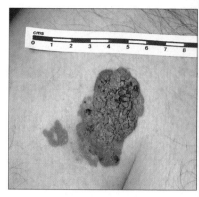

Fig. 5.47 Warty Bowen's disease

Sometimes an intra-epidermal squamous cell carcinoma may become so warty that it looks like a seborrhoeic wart: a trap for the unwary.

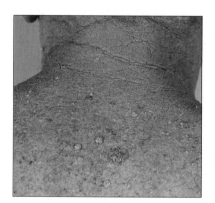

Fig. 5.48 Acanthosis nigricans

Velvety thickening of the skin in the flexures and around the neck is here accompanied by many lesions, some of which look like seborrhoeic keratoses, and others like skin tags. The commonest underlying cause is malignancy of the upper GI tract.

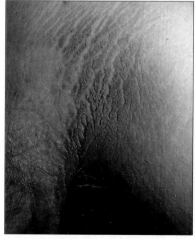

Fig. 5.49 Acanthosis nigricans

The rugose thickening of the axillary skin was one sign of this patient's insulin resistant diabetes.

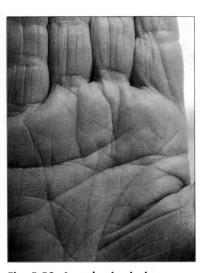

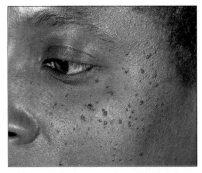

Fig. 5.51 Dermatosis papulosa migra
These small warty lesions on the face are common in those of Afro-Caribbean origin. Histologically they resemble seborrhoeic warts.

Fig. 5.50 Acanthosis nigricans
This patient had severe acanthosis nigricans and gastric carcinoma. Her palms were thickened, velvety and lined. An extreme version is known as a 'tripe palm'.

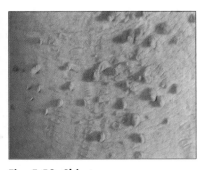

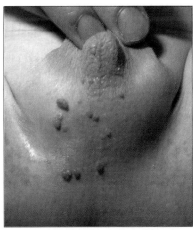

Fig. 5.52 Skin tags
These are common around the neck and in the major flexures of normal individuals. Here the profuse tags are associated with stretch marks in obesity. Skin tags are also a feature of tuberous sclerosis, acanthosis nigricans, acromegaly and diabetes.

Fig. 5.53 Molluscum contagiosum
This boy's parents were surprised to see skin tags appearing in his groin. They were, in fact, the lesions of molluscum contagiosum, each showing the typical central umbilication. Mollusca may become pedunculated in the flexures of children.

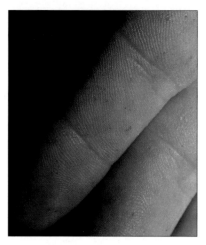

Fig. 5.54 Punctate keratoses
Not dirt but punctate keratoses. They also
affected the palms and ran as an
autosomal dominant trait in the family.

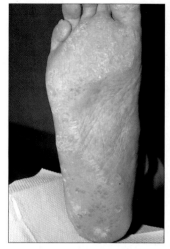

Fig. 5.55 Arsenical keratoses
Keratoses of the palms and soles
are a reminder of the arsenical
tonic taken by this patient for
several years. His risk of developing
an internal carcinoma remains high.

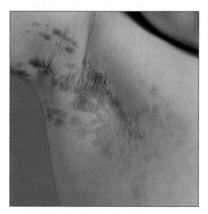

Fig. 5.56 Epidermal naevus
This lesion, present since birth, shows the
characteristic linearity of an epidermal
naevus and follows Blaschko's lines down
the arm and around the chest. Such
lesions are due to cutaneous mosaicism.

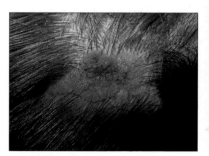

Fig. 5.57 Sebaceous naevus
At birth just a flat hairless area, at puberty
it became obviously yellow and raised as
the abnormal sebaceous glands responded
to increasing levels of circulating
androgen. These lesions may develop
basal cell carcinomata in adult life.

Chapter 6

Colours

Hyperpigmentation is not always due to an excess of melanin (Fig. 6.1), or hypopigmentation to its lack. Colour changes in the skin are often subtle and require natural light for their detection. In addition a liability to develop pigmentary abnormalities, and the importance of these, varies from race to race.

HYPERPIGMENTATION

LOCALIZED

An excess of pigmented lesions should raise suspicions of an associated internal disorder. More than six café au lait patches (Figs. 6.2 and 6.3), for example, suggest **neurofibromatosis**. The pigmented lesions of the **McCune–Albright syndrome** are larger and have a more irregular outline (Fig. 6.4); other features include polyostotic fibrous dysplasia and endocrine abnormalities such as precocious puberty. The whorled lesions of **incontinentia pigmenti** (Fig. 10.5) follow Blaschko's lines (Fig. 2.34): mental retardation and skull, palatal and dental abnormalities may be present. Pigmentation in a **chimera** takes up a checker-board pattern (Fig. 6.5).

Lentigines (Fig. 6.6) are brown macules, less than 1 cm in diameter, and usually an innocent finding, becoming more numerous with age. Occasionally they are a marker for internal disease. In the **Peutz–Jeghers syndrome** (Figs. 6.7 and 6.8), lentigines on and around the lips are associated with intestinal polyps which occasionally turn malignant. In the **Cronkite-Canada syndrome**, multiple lentigines on the backs of the hands may also be associated with gastrointestinal polyposis.

The acronym of the '**LEOPARD**' **syndrome** stands for **L**entiginosis with cardiac abnormalities demonstrated by ECG, **O**cular hypertelorism, **P**ulmonary stenosis, **A**bnormal genitalia, **R**etardation of growth and **D**eafness. **Centrofacial lentiginosis** is also associated with internal abnormalities: small brown or black lentigines appear in a horizontal band on the centre of the face during the first years of life — the association is with spina bifida and epilepsy.

Melanocytic naevi may be congenital (Figs. 1.57 and 6.9) or acquired (Fig. 1.58). The risk of developing malignant melanoma increases in those with giant congenital melanocytic naevi, the atypical mole syndrome (Fig. 6.10) or multiple acquired melanocytic naevi.

Freckling and lentiginosis are early features of **xeroderma pigmentosum** (Figs. 8.22–8.23): later the picture is dominated by multiple skin tumours. Basal cell carcinomas, as well as malignant melanomas, may be heavily pigmented (Fig. 1.64). The stuck-on appearance of the common pigmented seborrhoeic keratosis (Figs. 5.45 and 5.46) is easy to identify.

Skin inflammation is often followed by **post-inflammatory hyperpigmentation**. This may be a striking feature of resolving lichen planus (Fig. 5.15), of fixed drug eruptions (Fig. 6.11, 1.116 and 4.89) and of atopic eczema (Fig. 6.12). **Melasma** (Fig. 6.13) is often associated with the use of oral contraceptives.

GENERALIZED

A **diffuse hypermelanosis** may accompany severe ill-health, whatever its cause. This is particularly obvious in **malabsorption**, **chronic renal failure**, and in the cachectic stage of **malignant disease**; an even more striking melanosis can be caused by a disseminated **melanoma**. The bronzed pigmentation of **haemochromatosis** (Fig. 6.14) is associated with diabetes and liver disease. A deep tan is seen in **Nelson's syndrome** in patients with Cushing's disease treated by bilateral adrenalectomy, and with other ACTH producing tumours, such as an oat-cell carcinoma of the bronchus. However, pigmentation is not a feature of Cushing's syndrome itself. In **Addison's disease**, the pigmentation is most marked in exposed areas, scars and skin creases (Fig. 6.15), on the genitals and in the mouth (Fig. 4.44).

Several **drugs** also cause a characteristic hyperpigmentation. That due to phenothiazines has a slate-grey colour (Fig. 6.16) and to amiodarone a silver-grey hue (Fig. 6.17). Both are most obvious on exposed areas. Long-term chloroquine usage both bleaches the hair and pigments the skin. Other important drug causes of skin pigmentation include minocycline (Figs. 6.18 and 6.19) and busulphan.

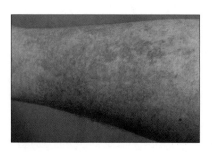

Fig. 6.1 Benign capillaritis
This gingery colour is typical of haemosiderin rather than melanin. Fragile capillaries on the lower leg create a fine dusting of petechiae: the purple colour of which fades and turns brown as haemoglobin changes into haemosiderin.

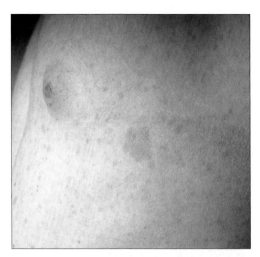

Fig. 6.2
Neurofibromatosis
An early stage, with many
small and one slightly larger
café au lait patch. Axillary
freckling is characteristic of
neurofibromatosis.

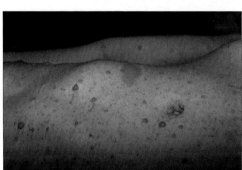

Fig. 6.3
Neurofibromatosis
Similar pigmented lesions, as
well as a scattering of small
neurofibromas.

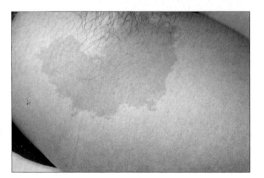

**Fig. 6.4 McCune–Albright
syndrome**
Large fawn patches, often with
a highly irregular edge, are
part of this syndrome. Other
features include polyostotic
fibrous dysplasia, endocrine
over-activity including
hyperthyroidism, and
precocious puberty.

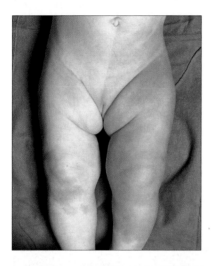

Fig. 6.5 Chimera
These are very rare, and usually detected by blood grouping because there are two populations of red cells. Patchy pigmentation may be of a checker-board type, with a sharp midline colour change.

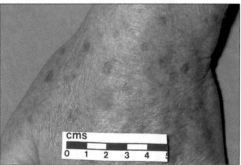

Fig. 6.6 Simple lentigines ('liver spots')
The back of this hand shows both the common macular, smooth-surfaced lentigines, due to longterm sun exposure, and the slightly raised areas with a matt-finish, probably a variant on the seborrhoeic wart theme.

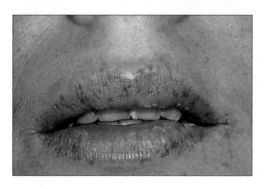

Fig. 6.7 Peutz–Jeghers syndrome
Pigmented macules occur on the lips and buccal mucosa. The internal association is with intestinal polyps, which may bleed or obstruct.

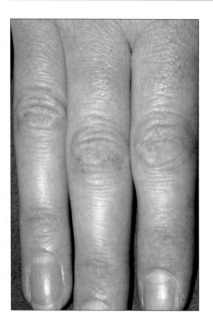

Fig. 6.8 Peutz–Jeghers syndrome
Subtle small lentigines may be seen on the
backs of the fingers in both the
Peutz–Jeghers and Cronkite–Canada
syndromes.

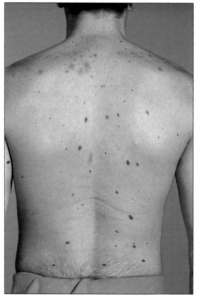

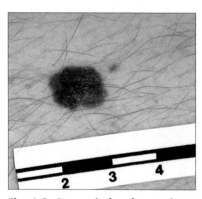

**Fig. 6.9 Congenital melanocytic
naevus**
Melanocytic naevi greater than one cm in
diameter are usually present or appear
shortly after birth. The risk of transformation
into malignant melanoma is small
compared with that for large lesions.

**Fig. 6.10 Atypical mole
syndrome**
A familial trait in which multiple, large
naevi carry an increased risk of
changing into a malignant melanoma.
Note the irregular shapes, sizes and
degree of pigmentation.

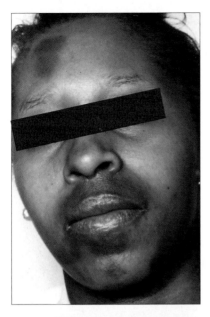

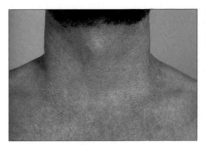

Fig. 6.12 Atopic eczema
This rippled pattern of hyperpigmentation around the neck is characteristic of chronic severe widespread atopic eczema.

Fig. 6.11 Fixed drug eruption
These ugly areas of hyperpigmentation represent the quiet stage of a fixed drug eruption secondary to phenolphthalein in a laxative. When the medication is taken, the areas become inflamed and swollen.

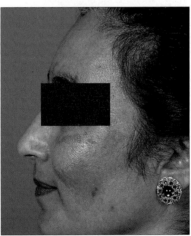

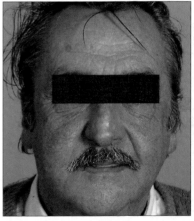

Fig. 6.13 Melasma (Chloasma)
A normal accompaniment of pregnancy, melasma can also be induced by oral contraception plus exposure to sunlight.

Fig. 6.14 Haemochromatosis
This patient had the full triad of diabetes, cirrhosis of the liver and bronzed discolouration. The pigmentation is due both to melanin and iron deposition.

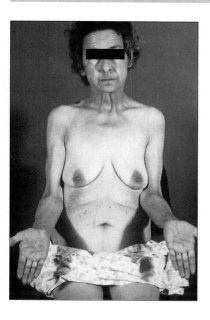

Fig. 6.15 Addison's disease
Increased pigmentation is obvious on exposed areas and in the palmar creases.

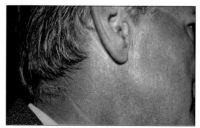

Fig. 6.16 Drug induced hyperpigmentation
This striking pigmentation was due to longterm phenothiazine therapy. Note the sparing of the skin protected from the light by his spectacles, by his ear, and in the creases.

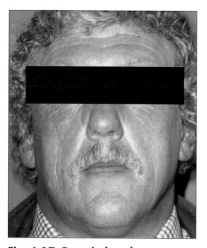

Fig. 6.17 Drug induced hyperpigmentation
Most patients on amiodarone accept this as a side effect of prolonged therapy.

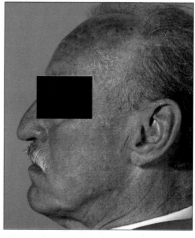

Fig. 6.18 Drug induced hyperpigmentation
Minocycline taken in high dose, longterm, for a trivial rosacea caused this facial pigmentation.

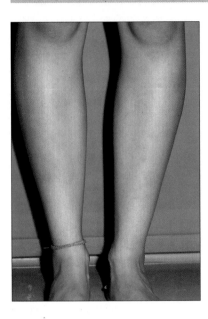

Fig. 6.19 Drug induced hyperpigmentation
Minocycline pigmentation can also be seen away from the face, as in this example of bluish-grey discolouration of the shins.

HYPOPIGMENTATION

LOCALIZED

Sharply defined white patches with no scaling but with some surrounding hyperpigmentation are likely to be due to **vitiligo**, in Caucasoids (Fig. 6.20). Spotty follicular repigmentation may be seen. Vitiligo often favours the skin around the eyes, nostrils, mouth, ears, nipples, urethra and anus, the fronts of the knees, backs of the hands, and wrists and the neck. There may be a family or personal history of vitiligo and of other autoimmune diseases. However, the segmental type of vitiligo has no association with autoimmunity. An area of symmetrical and total depigmentation occasionally appears around a banal melanocytic naevus. Such a **halo naevus** (Fig. 6.21) is benign, and the naevus in the centre often involutes spontaneously before the halo repigments. There may be vitiligo elsewhere.

Piebaldism is present at birth. Those affected have a white forelock (Fig. 4.17) and roughly symmetrical patches of depigmentation on the chest, abdomen and limbs. The Waardenburg syndrome also includes a white forelock, as well as separation of the medial epicanthic folds, prominent inner thirds of the eyebrows, irides of different colour and deafness.

Hypopigmented patches are seen in tuberculoid and some borderline types of **leprosy** (Figs. 6.22 and 6.23). Features which distinguish this from vitiligo include hypo-aesthesia, diminished hair and sweating within lesions, induration and an elevated edge. Local nerves may be thickened.

Pityriasis versicolor, although common, is not always recognized. It is due to overgrowth of the commensal yeast pityrosporum orbiculare. Its macules have a branny scaling and are fawn against an untanned background but pale when the surrounding skin is tanned (Fig. 6.24).

A **naevus anaemicus** (Fig. 6.25) is a localized area of increased vascular reactivity to catecholamines. They are most common on the trunk. When rubbed, the surrounding skin, but not the pale area itself, becomes pinker. The association here is with neurofibromatosis.

'Ash leaf' depigmented macules occur in 80% of those with **tuberous sclerosis** (Figs. 1.59, 1.60, 5.29 and 4.76). They may be its only manifestation at birth. Their detection is made easier by Wood's (ultraviolet) light. Other features include adenoma sebaceum, cerebral glioma, epilepsy, mental retardation, periungual fibromata, retinal abnormalities, connective tissue naevi, and renal and heart tumours.

Some consider that **lichen sclerosus et atrophicus** (Figs. 6.26, 6.27 and 4.81–4.83) is a variant of localized scleroderma (morphoea). Most common in women, the white shiny and atrophic macules, with follicular accentuation, occur at the base of the neck, over the shoulder blades, below the breasts and around the vulva and anus.

GENERALIZED

Phenylketonuria, an autosomal recessive trait, is a rare cause of hypopigmentation. Fair skin and hair are accompanied by photosensitivity and often by atopic eczema. The subtle skin changes of **hypopituitarism** are atrophy, pallor and a yellow tinge. Sexual hair is thinned or lost.

The entire skin is white and pigment is lacking in the hair, iris and retina in **oculocutaneous albinism** (Fig. 4.16). One type is due to a defect in tyrosinase, the most important enzyme in melanin synthesis. Albinos have poor sight, photophobia and rotatory nystagmus. Some are tyrosinase positive and have a little pigment in their skin, iris and hair as well as freckles. Albinos in the tropics develop skin tumours in early life.

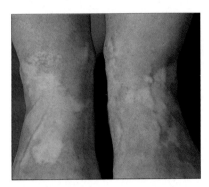

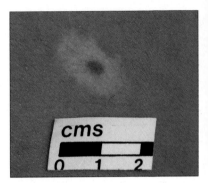

Fig. 6.20 Vitiligo
These symmetrical sharply defined areas of depigmentation are surrounded by skin which is hyperpigmented. The pale areas burn easily in the sun. Vitiligo is found more commonly than by chance in a number of autoimmune disorders including thyroid disease, pernicious anaemia, Addison's disease and diabetes mellitus.

Fig. 6.21 Halo naevus
A vitiligo-like patch appears around a banal melanocytic naevus. In this case the naevus became flatter, pinker, and eventually disappeared after several years. Vitiligo may be present elsewhere.

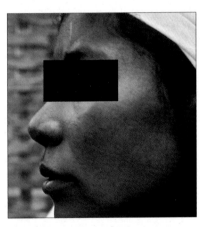

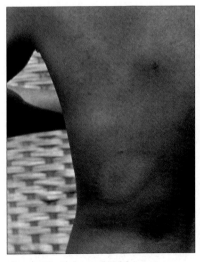

Fig. 6.22 Tuberculoid leprosy
Hypopigmentation may be a feature of all types of leprosy but is particularly obvious at the tuberculoid end of the spectrum. Sensory impairment and thickening of adjacent nerves should be looked for.

Fig. 6.23 Tuberculoid leprosy
The depigmented lesions on this patient's back were hypo-aesthetic.

Fig. 6.24 Pityriasis versicolor

This condition appears as pale, slightly scaly areas against a sun-tanned background, and as fawn areas against a pale skin. The scaly areas are due to overgrowth of commensal pityrosporum yeasts. Occasional medical associations include Cushing's disease and possibly AIDS.

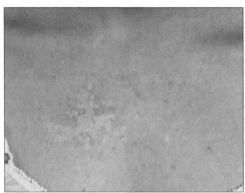

Fig. 6.25 Naevus anaemicus

This pale area has been rubbed and has failed to turn red whereas the surrounding normal skin has done so. This is a biochemical naevus in which the affected capillaries constrict abnormally in response to normal circulating levels of catecholamines. These lesions may be an isolated abnormality or occur with neurofibromatosis.

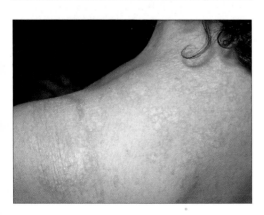

Fig. 6.26 Lichen sclerosus et atrophicus

This is characterized by non-indurated white shiny macules, sometimes with obvious follicular plugging. The most common and important site of involvement is the vulva (Figs. 4.81 and 4.82), where the condition may be a precursor of carcinoma. Another typical site is the area of pressure under a bra-strap and on the upper back, as seen here.

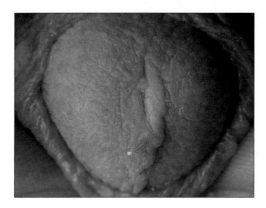

Fig. 6.27 Lichen sclerosus et atrophicus Involvement of the male urethral meatus may cause stenosis and difficulty with the passage of urine. In addition the foreskin may become adherent to the glans.

OTHER COLOURS

Changes in skin colour are important but easily missed. For example, haemoglobin has to drop below 8g/dl before **anaemia** can be reliably detected. In pernicious anaemia the skin has an added lemon yellow tinge.

Mild **jaundice** is hard to detect in artificial light. The sclera is a good place to look (Fig. 6.28). In longstanding jaundice, the skin takes on a bronzed colour, as in primary biliary cirrhosis, where pruritus is marked and scratch marks are common. **Green discolouration** may be a sign of opportunistic infection by pseudomonas aeruginosa (Fig. 6.29).

The differential diagnosis of yellow skin includes **carotenaemia** (Fig. 6.30) and **mepacrine** therapy. **Xanthomas** have a characteristic yellow colour too (Figs. 6.31 and 6.32); an underlying hyperlipidaemia should be sought.

Many patients with chronic **renal failure**, particularly those on dialysis, develop a muddy yellow/brown colour. The blue-black colour of **ochronosis** (alkaptonuria), is most easily seen where cartilage lies close to the surface, as on the ears.

The selection of pigments used by **tattoo artists** (Figs. 6.33 and 6.34) includes: black (carbon), blue (cobalt salts), brown (iron salts), green (chrome salts), yellow (cadmium sulphide), and red (cinnabar or vegetable dye). Medical associations are linked to promiscuity and drug addiction.

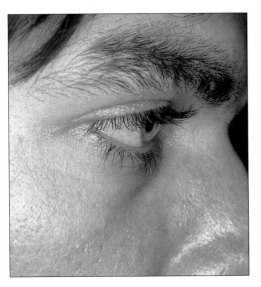

Fig. 6.28 Jaundice
This is seen most easily on the ocular sclerae. In this it differs from carotenaemia which is most obvious where the keratin layer is thick as on the palms and soles.

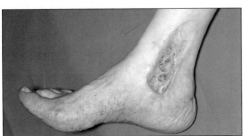

Fig. 6.29 Pseudomonas aeruginosa infection
The colour and smell of this ulcer pointed to an opportunistic infection by pseudomonas aeruginosa.

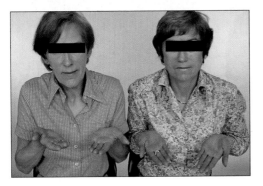

Fig. 6.30 Carotenaemia
These sisters took beta-carotene for their familial type of proto-porphyria. The orange colour is most obvious on the palms, where the stratum corneum is thickest.

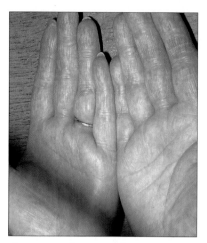

Fig. 6.31 Plane xanthomas
Yellow palmar creases are well seen here.
This type of plane xanthoma is characteristic
of type III hyperlipoproteinaemia.

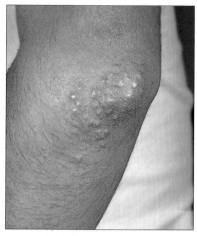

Fig. 6.32 Tuberous xanthomas
The yellowish colour is the clue to the
diagnosis here, investigation for
underlying hyperlipidaemia is essential.

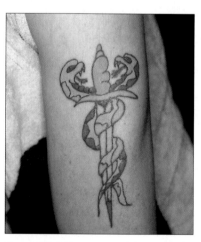

Fig. 6.33 Tattoo A tasteful mixture of
pigments (black due to carbon, light blue
due to cobalt, green due to chromium
salts, yellow due to cadmium, red due to
mercury or vegetable dyes).

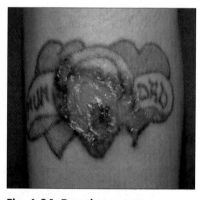

Fig. 6.34 Reaction to tattoo
Allergic reactions to individual pigments
are confined to areas of one particular
colour. Here the reaction straddles areas
of various colours. Sarcoidosis should be
considered. Similarly, lichen planus and
psoriasis may occur as a Koebner
response in tattoos.

Chapter 7

Textures

The word texture is hard to define. However, even though looking at the skin will reveal a great deal, all dermatologists know that they can easily make diagnostic mistakes if asked to pronounce on the surface appearance alone of even quite banal eruptions. They derive extra and often crucial information from touching the affected areas.

DRYNESS

Strictly speaking, skin is dry only when sweating is reduced. This is most striking in the various **anhidrotic ectodermal dysplasias** (Fig. 7.1) which may predispose to heat exhaustion. The important clue is a failure to develop other ectodermal structures (hair, nails and teeth).

In contrast, the rough scaly skin of **ichthyosis** is due not to a lack of sweating, but to abnormal cells in the horny layer which flake off in clumps rather than individually. Increased water loss caused by this defective horny layer contributes to dryness. Each of the many sub-types of ichthyosis is likely to have its own genetic and biochemical defect (Fig. 7.2) but so far few of these have been delineated. Perhaps the most striking is the lack of steroid sulphatase in the severe X-linked recessive type of ichthyosis (Fig. 7.3). An acquired ichthyosis may occur in response to an underlying lymphoma.

The word **xerosis** describes a dry flakiness of the skin in the elderly, often accompanied by itching and most obvious in the winter. Xerosis predisposes to **asteatotic eczema** (Figs. 7.4 and 7.5). A general dryness of the skin may also be found in atopic eczema, in chronic renal or liver failure, in AIDS, in myxoedema, and in malabsorption, particularly of vitamin A or zinc. Localized dryness and cracking of the skin of the soles of the feet is seen in some atopic children (Fig. 7.6).

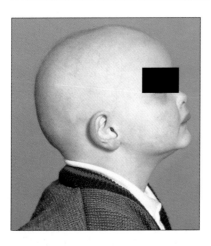

Fig. 7.1 Hypohidrotic ectodermal dysplasia
Sparse hair, abnormal nails, and reduced sweating are inherited as an X-linked recessive trait. Complications include hyperpyrexia, and recurrent chest infections. The typical pointed teeth of this condition are shown in Fig. 4.49.

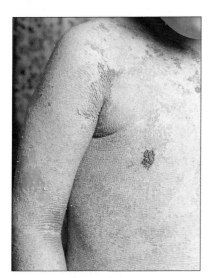

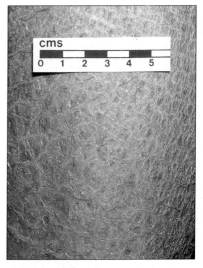

Fig. 7.2 Bullous ichthyosis (Siemens)
A rare condition characterized by very superficial blisters and desquamation, as seen on the arm as well as by generalized dry hyperkeratosis. This condition is due to a mutation of a keratin gene.

Fig. 7.3 Ichthyosis
This severe X-linked type of ichthyosis is due to a deficiency of steroid sulphatase. The large brown scales appear shortly after birth and involve the flexures. The condition persists throughout life. Corneal opacities and cryptorchidism may also be found.

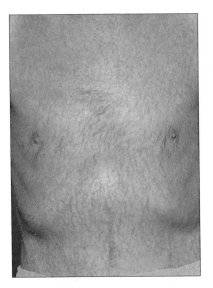

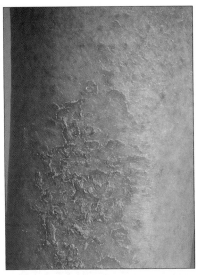

Fig. 7.4 Widespread asteatosis
This may sometimes be associated with zinc deficiency and sometimes occurs in chronic alcoholism.

Fig. 7.5 Asteatotic eczema
The splits in the stratum corneum are well shown. This itchy condition occurs during the winter in patients with dry skin. Diuretics predispose to it.

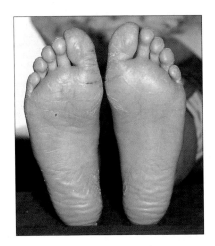

Fig. 7.6 Juvenile plantar dermatosis
Shiny dry weight bearing areas, accompanied by severe cracking, are seen on the feet of some atopic children. Walking becomes painful and difficult. The condition may be a reaction to modern shoe insole ingredients.

SWEATY SKIN

In **hyperhidrosis**, the superficial layers of the epidermis become white and macerated. Excessively sweaty palms and soles become livid, macerated and smelly due to bacterial colonization. **Pitted keratolysis**, a moth-eaten appearance of the soles, occurs in this setting (Fig. 7.7). Local hyperhidrosis of this kind plagues young adults and though **thyrotoxicosis** (Fig. 7.8), **acromegaly** (Fig. 7.14) and **anxiety states** should always be considered, no cause can usually be found.

Miliaria is due to blockage of eccrine sweat ducts. Invariably it is associated with heat intolerance. Similarly, **Fox–Fordyce disease** is due to the rupture and plugging of apocrine ducts, leading to the development of itchy, skin coloured papules in the axillae and other areas where apocrine glands are found (breasts, vulva).

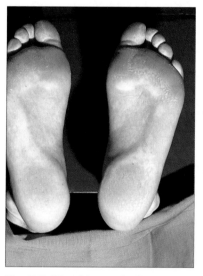

Fig. 7.7 Pitted keratolysis
Occlusive army boots plus sweaty feet lead to the overgrowth of commensal diphtheroids. These digest keratin and liberate a characteristic unpleasant smell.

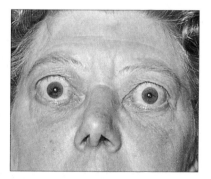

Fig. 7.8 Thyrotoxicosis
No marks for missing this patient's remediable cause of hyperhidrosis.

GREASY SKIN

A high sebum secretion rate is physiological in teenagers and a prerequisite for the development of **acne** (Fig. 7.9). Increased sebum secretion is also found in **acromegaly** (Fig. 7.14) and **Parkinson's disease**. **Senile sebaceous hyperplasia** (Fig. 7.10) is common on elderly faces.

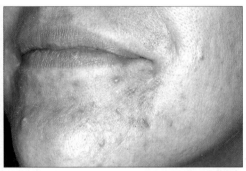

Fig. 7.9 Seborrhoea
This is a typical accompaniment of teenage acne, here of the small papule variety.

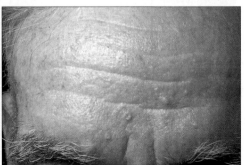

Fig. 7.10 Senile sebaceous hyperplasia
This patient had a greasy skin all his life and has now developed papular lesions on his forehead. They have a central depression and a raised yellowish rim. They are often mistaken for basal cell carcinomas.

THICK SKIN

Any of the skin's layers can become thick.

THE STRATUM CORNEUM

This is greatly increased in the various patterns of inherited **palmo-plantar keratoderma** (Fig. 7.11) which are usually isolated abnormalities, due to mutations in keratin genes. **Post-menopausal keratoderma** (Fig. 10.10) looks similar, but seems to be a response to hormonal changes in some post-menopausal women. It can easily be mistaken for **hyperkeratotic eczema** or **psoriasis** (Fig. 7.12). Scalp hairs impede the shedding of scales and untreated scalp psoriasis, in particular, can become raised and bumpy.

THE EPIDERMIS AS A WHOLE

Lichenification is a leathery thickening in which the normal skin markings are more obvious than usual. It is a response to scratching and rubbing and is most striking in atopic dermatitis (Fig. 7.13). The velvety thickening and pigmentation of the flexures of **acanthosis nigricans**, and its internal associations, are shown in Figs. 5.48–5.50.

THE DERMIS

Obvious internal causes are responsible for the thick skin of **acromegaly** (Fig. 7.14) and **thyroid acropachy**. Some **connective tissue naevi** (Fig. 7.15) are associated with osteopoikilosis (Fig. 7.16). The skin is hard and thick both in localized (Fig. 7.17) and systemic (Figs. 7.18–7.20) **scleroderma**, and in the **lipodermatosclerosis** of post-phlebetic legs (Fig. 7.21). The skin on the fingers of some **diabetics** may be tight enough to restrict movement (Fig. 7.22). The skin also thickens if the dermis is infiltrated with cells, as in the generalized type of cutaneous **mastocytosis** (Fig. 7.23), or if abnormal materials are deposited in it. Cutaneous **amyloidosis** (Figs. 7.48 and 7.49) may be associated with multiple myeloma; **scleromyxoedema** (Fig. 1.46) with paraproteinaemia; and the **muco-polysaccharidoses** with a variety of problems including mental defect and cardiac involvement. **Pretibial myxoedema** (Fig. 7.46) of thyroid origin can be closely mimicked by the thickened 'mossy' skin of chronic **lymphoedema** of the legs (Fig. 7.47); the arms can also be affected (Fig. 7.24). There is even a current school of thought which links rosacea and **rhinophyma** (Fig. 7.25) with helicobacter pylori infection.

THE SUBCUTANEOUS FAT

Some thickening is a normal accompaniment of ageing. 'Michelin tyre' babies with diffuse fat hypertrophy are rare.

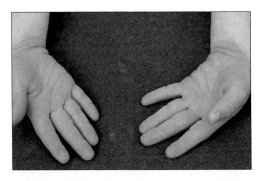

Fig. 7.11 Tylosis
Usually inherited as an autosomal dominant trait. An association with oesophageal carcinoma is disproportionately well known but found only in three families.

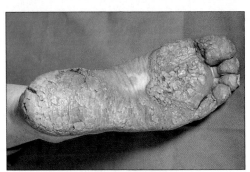

Fig. 7.12 Psoriasis
Although the picture is dominated here by gross hyperkeratosis, these changes are due to psoriasis and marginated red areas are seen on the insteps.

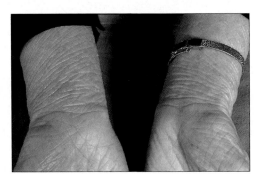

Fig. 7.13 Lichenification
This leathery response to scratching shows an increase in skin markings, here seen in a patient with atopic eczema of the flexor aspect of the wrists.

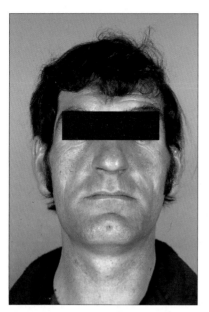

Fig. 7.14 Acromegaly
The skin is greasy and thick. The features
are coarse and there is frontal bossing.

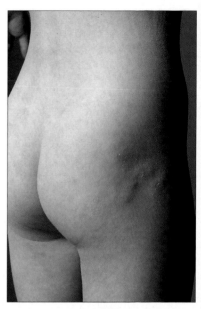

Fig. 7.15 Connective tissue naevi
Often hard to see, hence the need for
side-lighting. Always bear in mind
tuberous sclerosis and osteopoikilosis.

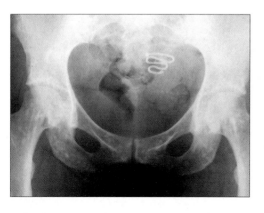

Fig. 7.16 Osteopoikilosis
Many small opacities can be
seen in the femoral heads and
in the pelvic bones. The
combination with connective
tissue naevi is known as the
Buschke–Ollendorf syndrome.

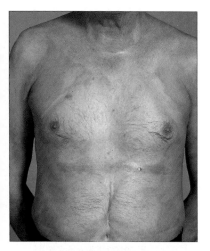

Fig. 7.17 Morphoea
This form of scleroderma remains localized to the skin. These yellow tightly bound down areas, encircling the chest, were sufficient to cause respiratory difficulty.

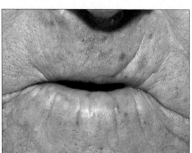

Fig. 7.18 Systemic sclerosis
This patient had much difficulty in forcing his false teeth into his mouth. Radial furrowing and telangiectasia are obvious.

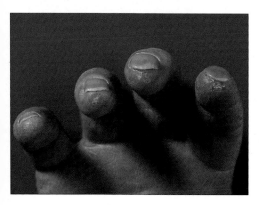

Fig. 7.19 Calcinosis in systemic sclerosis
This patient had the CREST variant. Whitish chalky material was regularly discharged from the finger tips; painful ulceration and loss of pulp tissue followed, together with beaking of the finger nails — most obvious here on the index and middle fingers.

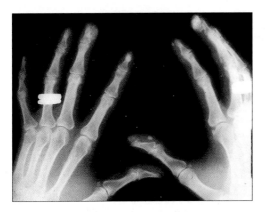

Fig. 7.20 Systemic sclerosis — calcinosis
Radio-opaque calcium deposits are seen in the pulps of the fingers and thumbs.

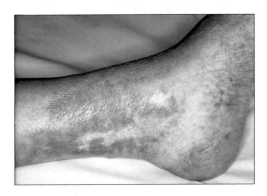

Fig. 7.21 Lipodermatosclerosis
Scarring, pigmentation and loss of hairs are due here to chronic venous hypertension.

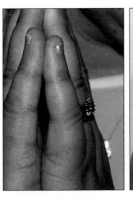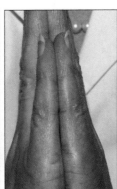

Fig. 7.22 Diabetic thick skin
The 'prayer test' demonstrates how the thick waxy skin of the fingers of a diabetic (on the left side) inhibits mobility as compared to normal fingers (seen on the right).

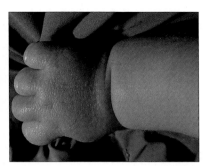

Fig. 7.23 Diffuse mastocytosis
The skin of this baby is diffusely infiltrated with mast cells, producing a thickened pig skin-like appearance. The bone marrow was also heavily infiltrated. Death from histamine shock is a real risk.

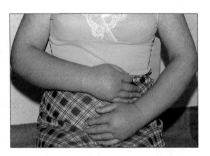

Fig. 7.24 Chronic lymphoedema
Recurrent bacterial infections originating in microvesicular eczema of the palms were responsible for these changes.

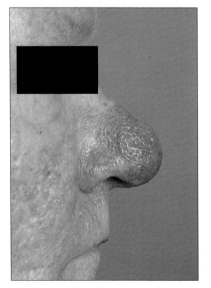

Fig. 7.25 Rhinophyma
Massive sebaceous gland hypertrophy is responsible for the very thick skin of the nose seen in this patient with rosacea.

THIN SKIN

Skin atrophy is due to a decrease in dermal connective tissue. **Ageing** is the most common cause (page 229) and it is most striking on uncovered skin exposed to longwave ultraviolet radiation. The combination of paper-thin skin (Fig. 7.26) and purpura, on the back of the hands of the elderly (Fig. 7.27), is a good example of this. Skin atrophy is also common in **rheumatoid disease**, especially in older patients.

Stretch marks are common in pregnancy (Fig. 10.8) but may also appear on the backs of rapidly growing teenagers (Fig. 7.28). Stretch marks may be seen in the wake of an infection of molluscum contagiosum (Fig. 7.32).

Glucocorticoids cause skin atrophy by depressing fibroblast activity. Thin skin and striae are therefore common in Cushing's syndrome and in patients on systemic steroids (Fig. 7.30). Strong topical steroids, especially if applied under occlusion, cause atrophy rapidly (Figs. 7.29 and 7.31).

Thick skin in diabetics (Fig. 7.22) has already been illustrated. Localised areas of atrophy, necrobiosis lipoidica (Fig. 7.33), are seen on the shins of about one percent of diabetics. Insulin injections may cause striking subcutaneous atrophy (Fig. 7.34).

Poikiloderma is the term used for a combination of atrophy, reticulate pigmentation and telangiectasia. It may be caused by X-irradiation. One form, **poikiloderma vasculare atrophicans** (Fig. 2.45), is a precursor of cutaneous T cell lymphoma. Paradoxically **morphoea** (Fig. 7.17) may resolve to leave atrophy of the skin and underlying tissues (Fig. 7.35).

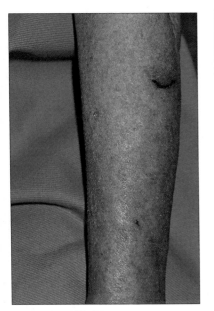

Fig. 7.26 Old skin
Minor trauma easily raises a typical crescentic flap, the edges of which become necrotic.

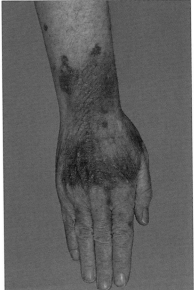

Fig. 7.27 Senile purpura
A thin skin with poorly supported dermal vessels which rupture with minor trauma. Coagulation studies will be normal.

Fig. 7.28 Stretch marks
Stretch marks are also common in normal adolescents. They are a response to rapid growth, and sometimes to sporting activities. Cushing's disease need not be suspected.

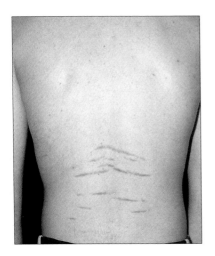

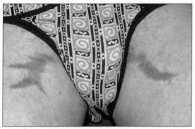

Fig. 7.29 Stretch marks
In this case the stag horn-shaped stretch marks were due to excessive topical corticosteroid applications rather than to systemic corticosteroid therapy.

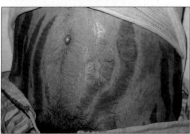

Fig. 7.30 Striae from systemic corticosteroid treatment
Gross in this patient and indistinguishable from those seen in Cushing's syndrome.

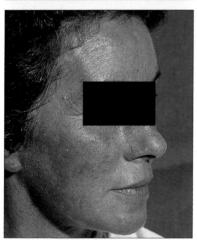

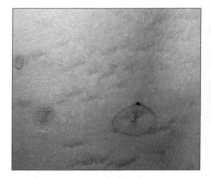

Fig. 7.31 Atrophy from topical corticosteroid applications
The mistaken use of strong topical cortico-steroid applications in a patient with rosacea has led to severe thinning of the skin with accompanying erythema and telangiectasia. Minimal hirsutism is also seen.

Fig. 7.32 Stretch marks
Stretch marks can sometimes be seen amongst molluscum contagiosum lesions. Here they are due to the local release of collagenase.

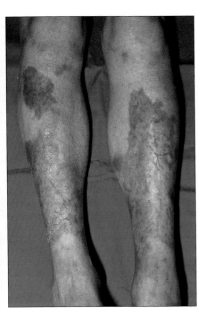

Fig. 7.33 Necrobiosis lipoidica
This is strongly associated with diabetes mellitus. Usually the diabetes comes first. The lesions lie on the shins. The surface of the skin becomes thin and shiny, telangiectasia can be seen and lesions often have a characteristic yellowish colour.

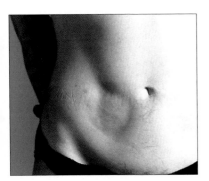

Fig. 7.34 Insulin lipoatrophy
The ugly area of fat-loss followed repeated insulin injections into the same area.

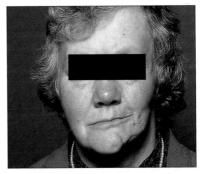

Fig. 7.35 Facial hemiatrophy
Atrophy involves the skin and subcutaneous tissues, but also the muscles and underlying bone. This condition may be the end result of localized scleroderma.

LAX SKIN

The skin hangs in redundant folds in **cutis laxa** (Fig. 7.36), a defect of elastic tissue. This may be inherited or a legacy of episodes of urticaria and angioedema, complement deficiency, lupus erythematosus, penicillin allergy, sarcoidosis, syphilis and multiple myeloma. Sufferers develop a 'bloodhound' appearance. Emphysema and cardiac abnormalities follow damage to internal elastic tissue.

Many types of **Ehlers–Danlos syndrome** (Figs. 7.37 and 7.38) are now recognized — all are inherited abnormalities of collagen metabolism. They show, to a varying degree, excessive skin elasticity, hyperextensibility of joints , fragility of the skin and blood vessels, easy bruising and ugly ('papyraceous') scars (Fig. 7.39). Complications include subluxation of joints, varicose veins in early life, a liability to develop hernias, kyphoscoliosis, aortic aneurysms and ruptured large arteries, and internal haemorrhages.

Pseudoxanthoma elasticum (Figs. 7.40–7.42) may be an autosomal dominant or a recessive trait, affecting elastin and probably collagen formation. The skin of the neck, axillae, and less often of other body folds, becomes loose and wrinkled and looks like a 'plucked chicken' with yellowish papules in the affected areas. **Angioid streaks** are seen in the retina (Fig. 4.31). Arterial involvement may lead to coronary, cerebrovascular or peripheral artery disease with hypertension, haemorrhage and thrombosis.

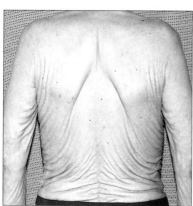

Fig. 7.36 Cutis laxa
Sagging skin folds give the appearance of premature ageing. Associated features may include herniae, diverticulae of the gut and bladder, hip dislocation and pulmonary emphysema.

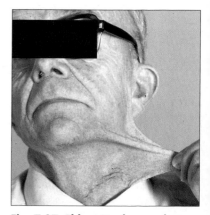

Fig. 7.37 Ehlers-Danlos syndrome
This patient's party-trick gives away the diagnosis.

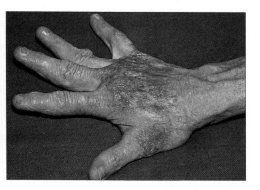

Fig. 7.38 Ehlers-Danlos syndrome
Vascular fragility leads to easy bruising. In children this may raise the mistaken diagnosis of physical abuse.

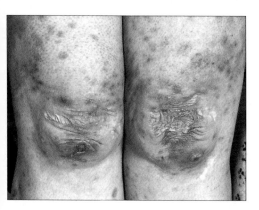

Fig. 7.39 Papyraceous scarring
This patient has Ehlers-Danlos syndrome. Complications depend on the type and include subluxation of joints, rupture of large arteries and aneurysms, eye haemorrhages, poor wound healing and atrophic scars.

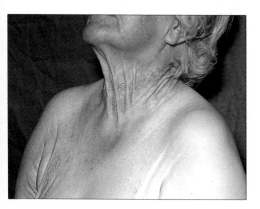

Fig. 7.40 Pseudoxanthoma elasticum
Plaques of small yellow papules are seen most often on the sides of the neck. The skin may be generally lax.

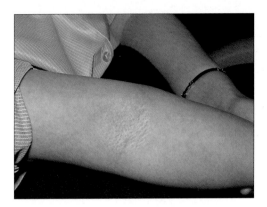

**Fig. 7.41
Pseudoxanthoma
elasticum**
Typical 'plucked chicken'
yellowish lesions in the bend
of an elbow.

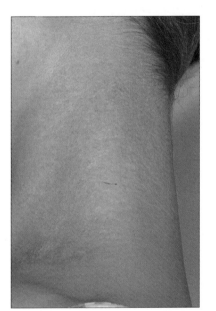

**Fig. 7.42 Pseudoxanthoma
elasticum**
Early and less obvious changes on the
side of the neck.

INFILTRATIONS AND DEPOSITS

Abnormal materials deposited in the skin may offer.clues to an underlying disease. **Gouty tophi**, for example, may be seen on the ears and finger tips (Figs. 7.43 and 7.44). The presence of **xanthomatous papules** or plaques (Figs. 6.31, 6.32 and 4.25) may be due to a primary hyperlipidaemia or secondary to diabetes mellitus, primary biliary cirrhosis, the nephrotic syndrome or hypothyroidism.

Deposits of **mucin** look like non-pitting oedema. In myxoedema (Fig. 7.45), the skin becomes puffy and the plaques of pretibial myxoedema (Fig. 7.46) have a peau d'orange appearance. This may be difficult to distinguish from chronic lymphoedema (Fig. 7.47).

In myelomatosis, waxy plaques of amyloid form most commonly around the eyes (Fig. 4.24). The appearance of the finger tips is characteristic in primary systemic amyloidosis (Fig. 7.48). The presence of 'pinch purpura' is also a good clue to amyloid deposition (Fig. 7.49).

The cutaneous deposits of **leukaemias** and **lymphomas** are erythematous macules or plaques (Figs. 1.74 and 1.75). **Metastases** from internal tumours are usually flesh coloured and may appear anywhere on the skin though tending to favour the scalp and the umbilicus (Figs. 1.79 and 1.80).

Calcium deposits are firm flesh coloured papules, nodules or plaques, usually on the extremities. Some are tender and ulcerate, discharging chalky material. The ulcers left are indolent and painful, especially on the finger tips (Fig. 7.19). Calcium deposition may be idiopathic but is often secondary to generalized disorders such as systemic sclerosis, pseudo-xanthoma elasticum and the Ehlers-Danlos syndrome. Metastatic calcification also occurs in hyperparathyroidism, sarcoidosis, carcinomatosis, Paget's disease, destructive bone disease and vitamin D excess (Fig. 7.50).

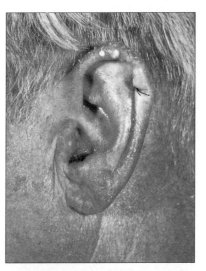

Fig. 7.43 Gouty tophi
The rim of the external ear is a classical site for the deposits of uric acid in tophaceous gout.

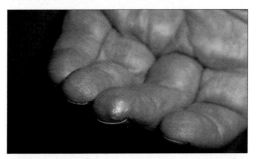

Fig. 7.44 Gouty tophi
Gouty tophi are also common on the finger tips.

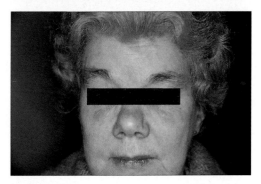

**Fig. 7.45
Hypothyroidism**
Severe hypothyroidism caused a moderate puffiness of the face, and slight thinning of the outer parts of her eyebrows but her scalp hair was not thinned.

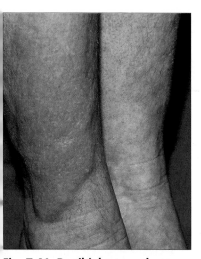

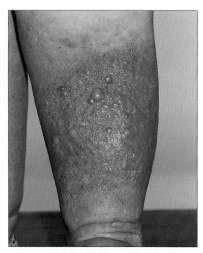

Fig. 7.46 Pretibial myxoedema
This patient's pretibial myxoedema began after the treatment of her exophthalmic thyrotoxicosis. The typical peau d'orange appearance is well known.

Fig. 7.47 Chronic lymphoedema
The inflamed irregular protuberances here were not related to thyroid disease but to chronic lymphoedema and repeated infections. Nevertheless, some excess of mucin was shown by special stains.

Fig. 7.48 Primary systemic amyloidosis
Soft, bulbous, infiltrated finger tips are typical. They bruise easily. No underlying myelomatosis was found here. Amyloidosis secondary to chronic disorders, such as rheumatoid arthritis or tuberculosis, seldom affects the skin.

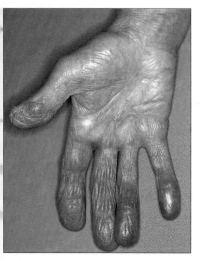

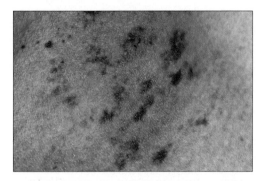

Fig. 7.49 Primary systemic amyloidosis
This patient presented with 'pinch purpura'. The walls of cutaneous blood vessels are infiltrated and rupture easily after trivial trauma, leading to purpuric areas of various sizes.

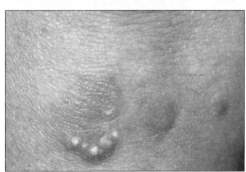

Fig. 7.50 Calcinosis circumscripta
No cause was ever found for these localised deposits of calcium salts in the skin. Serum calcium and phosphate were normal.

Chapter 8

Reactions

The skin protects us from many of the hazards in our environment. Its complex structure enables it to do this well but problems can still arise. Sometimes it becomes obvious from the history, and perhaps from the distribution of the rash, that environmental factors are important. This chapter covers some of the possibilities.

FLUSHING

Transient vasodilatation of the face, neck, chest and, occasionally, other parts of the body is common. **Physiological** flushing signals emotion (blushing (Fig. 8.1)), the menopause (hot flushes), or a reaction to spicy food.

Alcohol-induced flushing, is most common in Orientals. Disulfuram (Antabuse) and to a lesser extent chlorpropamide, worsen this. Other drugs which provoke flushing include nicotinic acid, nifedipine, and bromocriptine.

Flushing may be the first symptom of a **carcinoid tumour** (Fig. 8.2), either of gut origin which has metastasized to the liver, or a primary of the lung. Persistent facial erythema, scleroderma-like changes and a pellagra-like dermatitis occur later. Flushing, with episodic headache and palpitations, should arouse suspicion of a **phaeochromocytoma**. Flushing, headaches and palpitations may also be due to liberation of histamine in **mastocytosis**.

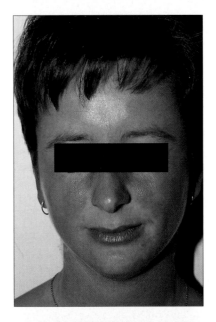

Fig. 8.1 Emotional flushing (blushing)
An embarassing remark is the usual cause. The reaction is the same in hot flushes, in reactions to spicy food and in drug-induced flushing.

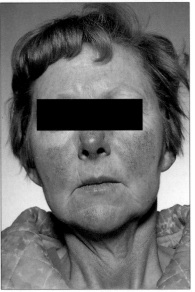

Fig. 8.2 Carcinoid syndrome
Recurrent episodes of flushing are followed eventually by a fixed telangiectatic dilatation of the blood vessels of the cheeks.

SCARRING

Damage to the dermis leads to scarring (Fig. 8.3). If the dermis is already abnormal, the resultant scar may be too; the papery scars of the **Ehlers–Danlos syndrome** (Fig. 7.39) are an example of this.

Characteristic scars are seen in **neurotic excoriations** (Fig. 8.4), **cicatricial pemphigoid** (Fig. 4.20), **herpes zoster**, **lupus vulgaris** (Fig. 8.5), **acne vulgaris** (Fig. 8.6), dystrophic **epidermolysis bullosa** (Fig. 8.7), **basal cell carcinoma** (Fig. 8.8) and **lupus erythematosus**. Implanted foreign material may discolour scars, as in the blue-black scars of coal miners.

Some factors predisposing to **keloid formation** (Figs. 8.9 and 8.10) are listed in Table 2.

The recognition of scarring, with loss of follicles, is important in the differential diagnosis of localized alopecia (page 93). **Stellate pseudoscars** (Fig. 8.11) follow the resolution of senile or steroid-induced purpura. Existing scars are favoured sites for cutaneous **sarcoidosis** (Fig. 8.12).

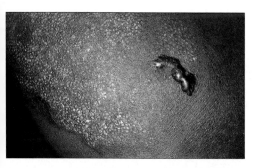

Fig. 8.3 Scarring after a burn
This slide shows a galaxy of changes including a keloid scar, areas of hyperpigmentation where the burn was least severe, and of hypopigmentation where it was most severe.

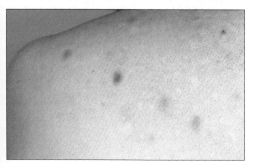

Fig. 8.4 Neurotic excoriations
The habit of picking at the skin in response to stress leads to a characteristic mixture of scabbed excoriations and whitish round scars.

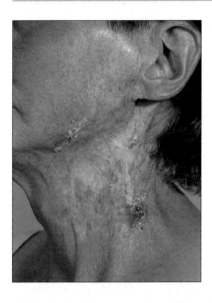

Fig. 8.5 Scarring following lupus vulgaris
An area of characteristic atrophic scarring, now showing a further complication. A squamous cell carcinoma has developed at the lower border of the scar and an early one on the angle of the jaw.

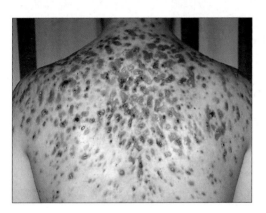

Fig. 8.6 Acne scarring
Disfiguring examples of this severity have become less common since the introduction of isotretinoin therapy.

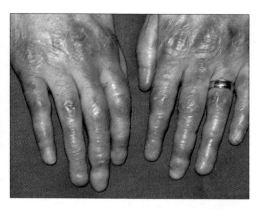

Fig. 8.7 Dystrophic epidermolysis bullosa
In this severe variant, blisters are followed by scars. Loss of nails is common.

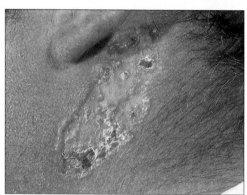

Fig. 8.8 Cicatricial basal cell carcinoma
This whitish area is a basal cell carcinoma which has excited a fibrous reaction. It may lack the pearly rim of the commoner types and requires a wider than usual excision.

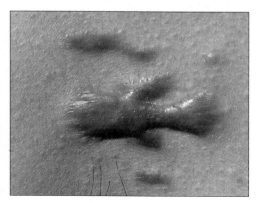

Fig. 8.9 Keloid
Typical lesions, running transversely across the front of the sternum, itself a favourite area for keloids.

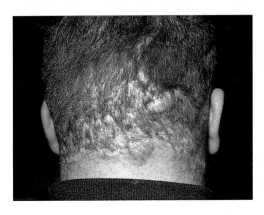

Fig. 8.10 Folliculitis keloidalis
Intractible inflammation and pustulation leads to thick areas of keloid formation: seen in males and perhaps related to ingrowing hairs encouraged by short hair styles.

Table 2
Factors predisposing to keloid formation

Afro-Caribbean origins

Site: upper trunk and earlobes

Family history of keloids

Burns, sepsis, foreign material

Wounds under tension

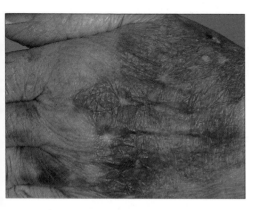

Fig. 8.11 Stellate pseudoscars
The whitish areas are pseudoscars, so called because the skin has never been broken. They follow the dispersion of senile purpura.

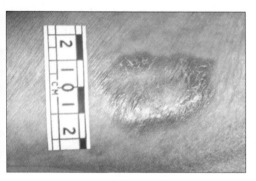

Fig. 8.12 Scar sarcoidosis
A thiny papery scar had been visible since a superficial injury several years previously. Its edge had recently become raised, pink and infiltrated by a sarcoid granuloma.

TO LIGHT

Sunburn is caused by wavelengths between 290–320nm (UVB) which do not penetrate window glass but reach the earth's surface on clear sunny days. Longer wavelengths (320-400nm, UVA) pass through glass but do not burn. A plentiful supply of UVA reaches the earth on bright but cloudy days.

Photosensitivity eruptions affect only exposed skin (Figs. 8.13 and 8.14) and spare areas such as the upper eyelids, below the nose and under the chin. The reaction itself (erythema, blistering, scaling, pigmentation, scarring, tumours) may offer a clue to the diagnosis. The problem may be familial, seasonal or drug-related.

A **drug cause** must be excluded first. Common culprits include amiodarone, chlorpropamide, nalidixic acid, oral contraceptives, phenothiazines (Fig. 6.16), psoralens (Fig. 8.15), quinidine, sulphonamides, tetracyclines and thiazides. Drug induced photosensitivity is usually provoked by UVA and reactions are usually like an exaggerated sunburn. Contact with some plants, for example giant hogweed, can lead to localized photosensitivity (Fig. 2.30).

Some conditions are made worse but not caused by ultraviolet radiation (UVR). These include **lupus erythematosus** (Fig. 1.23), **dermatomyositis** (Figs. 1.11 and 2.41), **pellagra** (Fig. 8.16), **cutaneous porphyrias, xeroderma pigmentosum** and **herpes simplex** infections (Fig. 1.112).

In **erythropoietic protoporphyria**, longwave UVA causes burning and pain on exposed skin, followed by oedema, thickening and scarring (Fig. 8.17). The skin signs of **cutaneous hepatic porphyria** (porphyria cutanea tarda) are fragility, hypertrichosis, pigmentation, and blisters or erosions on exposed skin (Figs. 8.18 and 8.19). Liver disease, usually from alcohol, but sometimes due to hepatitis or a hepatoma (Fig. 8.20), leads to an excess of uroporphyrins which are responsible for the photosensitivity. The urine is pink and fluoresces under Wood's (UVA) light (Fig. 8.21).

Xeroderma pigmentosum (Figs. 8.22 and 8.23) is due to a defect in DNA repair. Lentigines on exposed skin are soon followed by keratoses, squamous cell carcinomas, malignant melanomas and basal cell carcinomas.

Sunburn and **skin tumours** are common in widespread vitiligo (Fig. 6.20) and albinism (Fig. 4.16), especially in the tropics. In addition, in the elderly, elastosis (Fig. 8.24), actinic keratoses (Fig. 8.25), malignant melanomas, squamous cell carcinomas and to a lesser extent basal cell carcinomas are initiated by UVR exposure. The cause of some photosensitive disorders, including **polymorphic light eruption** and **chronic actinic dermatitis** (actinic reticuloid) is still unknown.

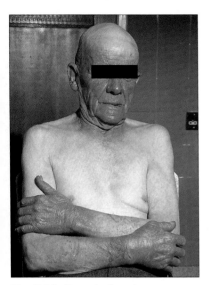

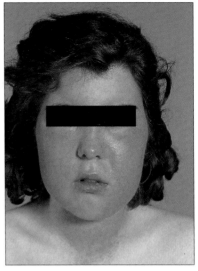

Fig. 8.13 Drug-induced photosensitivity
This patient regularly wore a cap which protected his scalp, and a shirt which protected his trunk and arms. A photosensitivity reaction, however, is well seen on his face and on the backs of his hands. The drug concerned was a thiazide diuretic.

Fig. 8.14 Photosensitivity
An unusually florid reaction with much oedema.

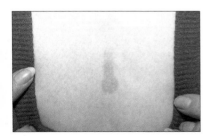

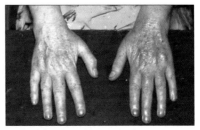

Fig. 8.15 Berloque dermatitis
The psoralen in a drop of perfume photosensitized this area, leaving striking pigmentation.

Fig. 8.16 Pellagra
The excessive response to sunlight, and residual tanning, were seen in an alcoholic with a nutritional deficiency of niacin.

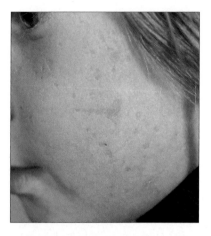

Fig. 8.17 Erythropoietic protoporphyria

This child reacts within a few minutes to sunlight. Burning and redness are followed by pitted scars, some of which are linear.

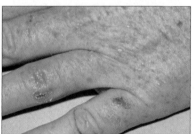

Fig. 8.18 Porphyria cutanea tarda

Features include skin fragility and a tendency to blister on exposed areas. Small blisters are seen on the little finger, and scattered milia indicate where blisters have formed in the past. Chronic alcoholism was the basis here.

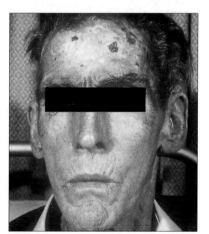

Fig. 8.19 Porphyria cutanea tarda — hepatoma

This alcoholic noticed that he was becoming excessively hairy and that the skin of his face was fragile and pigmented.

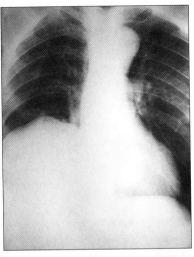

Fig. 8.20 Porphyria cutanea tarda — hepatoma
Same patient as in Fig. 8.19. Routine chest X-ray showed a raised right hemidiaphragm due to the hepatoma.

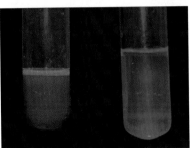

Fig. 8.21 Porphyria cutanea tarda — hepatoma
Same patient as in Figs. 8.19 and 20. Examination of a urine specimen under Wood's (ultraviolet-A) light showed a coral pink fluorescence in a chloroform extract of urine (left) due to excessive uroporphyrins. Normal urine on right.

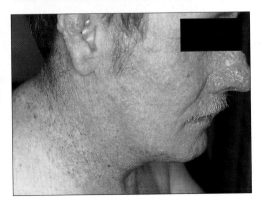

Fig. 8.22 Xeroderma pigmentosum
Several subtypes exist, all based upon an underlying inability to repair ultraviolet light induced DNA damage. The skin changes occur in early childhood and include atrophy, freckling and lentiginosis. Actinic keratoses and skin cancers, including melanomas, are common and life expectancy is much reduced.

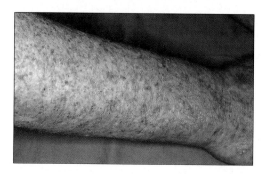

Fig. 8.23 Xeroderma pigmentosum
Severely damaged skin of the forearm.

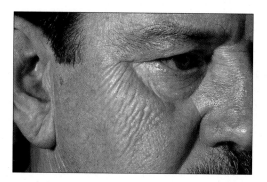

Fig. 8.24 Elastosis
Prolonged sun damage has caused this furrowed yellowish area of thickening on the cheek. Such areas often show many comedones, as is the case here.

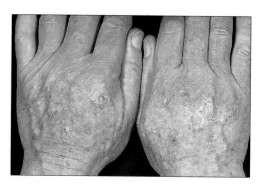

Fig. 8.25 Multiple actinic keratoses
These keratotic lesions are the result of heavy and prolonged exposure to sunlight in an outdoor worker. Only a few will evolve into a squamous cell carcinoma.

TO TRAUMA

The various types of **epidermolysis bullosa** share a tendency to develop blisters after minimal trauma. In the simplex types (Fig. 8.26), due to the presence of abnormal keratins, blisters arise above the basement membrane and heal without scarring. The dystrophic scarring types (Figs. 1.101, 1.102 and 8.7) are due to abnormalities of collagen VII, a major component of dermal anchoring fibrils.

Nikolski's sign (Fig. 8.27) is positive if finger pressure can force the superficial layers of the epidermis to separate from, and then slide sideways over the deeper layers. It occurs in **pemphigus** (Fig. 1.103) and in **toxic epidermal necrolysis** (Fig. 8.46) which is often drug induced. An abnormal pustular response to minor skin trauma, for example to venepuncture, is one feature of **Behçet's syndrome**. Those who have lichen planus or psoriasis may develop linear lesions in response to minor cuts or scratches. This is the **Koebner phenomenon** (Fig. 2.29).

Poorly supported dermal blood vessels rupture easily with minimal trauma. Senile or **steroid-induced purpura** (Fig. 8.11), the pinch purpura of systemic **amyloidosis** (Figs. 7.49 and 4.24), and the easy bruising of **scurvy**, are examples of this.

Sustained pressure over prominent bones may cause ischaemia and **pressure sores** (Fig. 8.28). Denervated skin is liable to develop **trophic ulcers** (Fig. 9.11). The skin is also unusually fragile in **porphyria cutanea tarda** (Fig. 8.18) and in the **Ehlers-Danlos syndrome** (Fig. 7.39). Minor pressure induces wheals, often linear, in those who are **dermographic** (Fig. 1.34). These appear immediately; but in **delayed pressure urticaria**, painful deep lesions appear hours after the pressure is applied. Repeated trauma from ill-fitting shoes may cause **onychogryphosis** (Fig. 8.29).

SELF-TRAUMA

Some patients damage their own skin, eg frank **dermatitis artefacta** (Fig. 8.30 and 2.28), **neurotic excoriations** (Figs. 8.31 and 8.32), and **localized neurodermatitis**. Those who pick at their acne may have few spots but many scabs and scars (Fig. 8.33). Other problems are due to minor habits of which the patient may be unaware: the ladder pattern of thumb nail ridging (Fig. 4.58) caused by **cuticle picking** is a good example of this. Some children annoy their parents by twisting and pulling out tufts of hair; an extreme form (**trichotillomania**) was responsible for the large areas of hair loss shown in Figure 8.34. Obsessionals who wash their hands too often may develop a chronic **irritant hand dermatitis** and chapping round the lips is often seen in atopic children who lick their lips as a nervous habit (Fig. 4.53). **Malingering** (Fig. 8.35) implies a conscious act, sometimes damaging to the skin, carried out to gain material advantage.

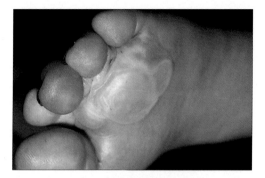

Fig. 8.26 Epidermolysis bullosa
A genodermatosis in which numerous large blisters are provoked by trivial friction, usually from shoes.

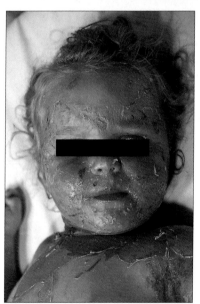

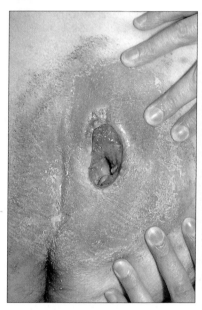

Fig. 8.27 Nikolski's sign
Here seen in an infant with staphylococcal scalded skin syndrome. The loosened epidermis slides sideways with minimal force — like wet wall-paper on a wall.

Fig. 8.28 Pressure sore
An advanced stage on the buttock of a patient confined to bed after a fractured neck of femur.

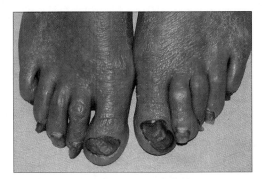

Fig. 8.29
Onychogryphosis
This thickening of the big toe nails is due to pressure from ill-fitting shoes.

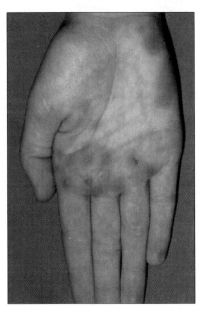

Fig 8.30 Dermatitis artefacta
An attempt by a young girl with multiple problems to draw attention to them by damaging her skin with a lighted cigarette.

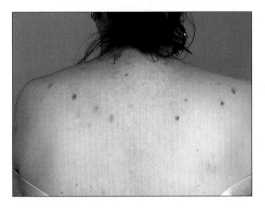

Fig. 8.31 Neurotic excoriations
This common reaction to stress consists of a mixture of scabbed, picked lesions and whitish scars. The habit is difficult to abolish.

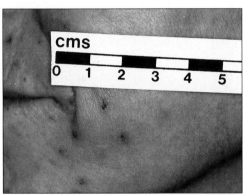

Fig. 8.32 Neurotic excoriations
Same patient as in Fig. 8.31. A close-up view of the typical picked lesions on the face. Some whitish scarring is seen along the angle of the jaw.

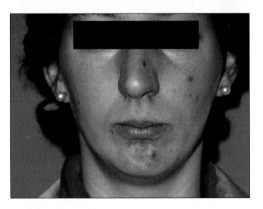

Fig. 8.33 Acne excoriée
The acne lesions themselves are often minor or invisible, in contrast to the excoriations produced by the patient's efforts to remove them. The habit is difficult to break and may lead to much scarring.

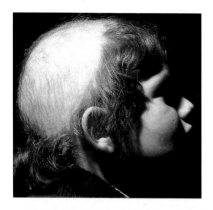

Fig. 8.34 Trichotillomania
This 'tonsure' pattern is the characteristic result of severe trichotillomania usually seen in teenage girls.

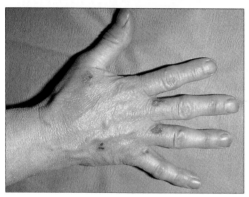

Fig. 8.35 Malingering
The rubbed and excoriated areas, between the fingers and elsewhere on the hand, were a deliberate attempt to obtain compensation under the guise of industrial dermatitis.

TO TEMPERATURE

COLD

Cold vasoconstricts and the skin then becomes pale. This effect is greater on veins than on arteries, whereas rewarming dilates arteries more, so that oedema occurs as arterial flow restarts. Cold can damage normal people, for example as **frostbite** in skiers (Figs. 1.98 and 8.36) or **trench foot** in soldiers. Other conditions, such as **chilblains** (Figs. 8.37 and 8.38), **acrocyanosis**, **erythrocyanosis**, **lupus pernio** (Fig. 8.39) and **livedo reticularis** (Fig. 2.42) are most common when skin blood flow is reduced by abnormal vessel tone, increased viscosity or platelet adhesiveness. Diseases to consider include **connective tissue disorders** (Fig. 8.40), **cryoglobulinaemia** (Figs. 8.41 and 8.42), **cold agglutininaemia** and the myeloproliferative diseases.

In **Raynaud's phenomenon**, paroxysmal attacks of sudden pallor of one or more digits are followed by cyanosis or erythema (Fig. 8.43). Usually idiopathic, particularly in young women, it may also be due to an underlying occlusive vascular disease, collagen vascular disease, cold agglutinins, cryoglobulinaemia or carcinoma. Exposure to occupational vibration, chemotherapy, smoking, and cyclosporin are other possible causes.

Occasionally **urticaria** is provoked by cold, for example by cold water or winds. Usually the cause cannot be identified; rarely cryoglobulins are found.

HEAT

Reactions to cold may be a useful indicator of systemic disease but reactions to heat are seldom significant. Patients with **rosacea** flush easily on entering a hot room. **Erythema ab igne** (Fig. 2.44) is sometimes seen in hypothyroidism. However, excessive sweating is usually not an over-reaction to heat.

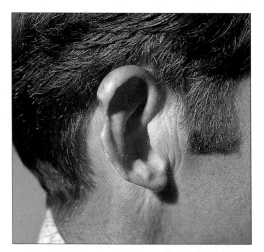

Fig. 8.36 Frostbite
A severe episode several years ago was responsible for this obvious loss of tissue from the rim of the ear.

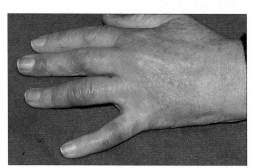

Fig. 8.37 Chilblains
The common type, as shown here, can be mimicked by chilblain lupus erythematosus and by sarcoidosis.

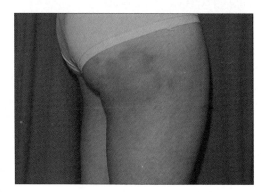

Fig. 8.38 Chilblains
Chilblains can affect areas other than the hands and feet. Typical lesions are seen on the outer thighs of those who ride horses under cold conditions.

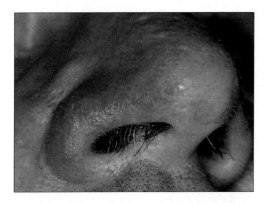

Fig. 8.39 Sarcoidosis (lupus pernio)

Bluish purple discolouration around the nostril which has not yet turned into a full blown lupus pernio. Nevertheless, the patient also had marked pulmonary sarcoidosis.

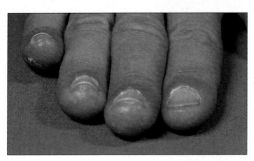

Fig. 8.40 Chilblain lupus erythematosus

Purplish perniotic lesions of the finger tips, with exacerbations during the winter. The patient did not develop systemic lupus erythematosus, although this sometimes happens.

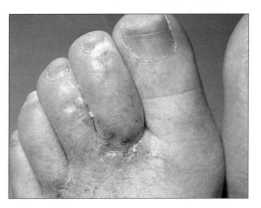

Fig. 8.41 Cryoglobulinaemia

Precipitation by cooling was followed by this unusual ulcer on the top of the foot. The condition may be secondary to myeloma, leukaemia or an autoimmune disease.

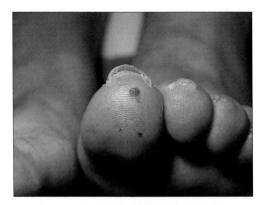

Fig. 8.42
Cryoglobulinaemia
Small purpuric lesions on cold extremities may also be due to cryoglobulinaemia.

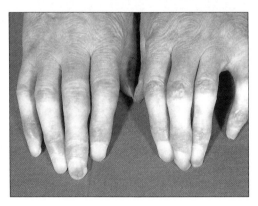

Fig. 8.43 Raynaud's disease
The most important underlying causes are connective tissue disorders such as systemic sclerosis (as in this patient) and lupus erythematosus.

TO TREATMENT

Skin reactions to **systemic drugs** are common and almost any drug can cause them. Some, for example penicillins, sulphonamides (Fig. 8.44), thiazides, phenylbutazone and allopurinol, seem especially prone to do so. Others, including digoxin, iron, vitamins and throxine, seldom cause problems. Doctors learn by experience into which category the drugs they prescribe fit. Although almost any drug can cause any eruption, some reactions occur most commonly with certain drugs (Table 3, Figs. 8.45–8.48). The main clues to a drug eruption include previous reactions to drugs, the introduction of the suspected drug just before the eruption appeared (Fig. 8.49), the recent prescription of a likely drug and the symmetrical nature of an eruption which fits with the track record of one of the current drugs.

Allergic contact dermatitis caused by topical medicaments is also common. Local antibiotics, antihistamines (Fig. 8.50), antiseptics and anaesthetics are the main culprits. Allergic contact dermatitis is one cause of a red swollen face and should be distinguished from erysipelas and angioedema.

Physical treatments may sometimes cause skin reactions. Psoriasis, lichen planus and viral warts may appear at the site of a recent surgical wound (Fig. 2.29). Sarcoidosis may involve longstanding scars. **Superficial X-ray therapy**, nowadays used for skin cancer in the aged, causes atrophy, scarring and telangiectasia (Fig. 8.51). Paradoxically, skin cancer is a late sequela (Fig. 8.52) and necrosis a late but rare complication. **Deep X-ray therapy** causes less dramatic skin changes but may induce localized scleroderma (Fig. 8.53). Prolonged ultraviolet **phototherapy** induces lentigines and skin cancer.

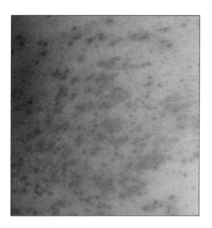

Fig. 8.44 Drug eruption
The common erythematous maculo-papular reaction, in this case due to a sulphonamide.

Table 3
Drug Eruptions and their Causes

Reaction Pattern	Drugs which Commonly Cause Reaction
Toxic erythema (Fig. 8.44)	Antibiotics, sulphonamides, thiazides, phenylbutazone
Urticaria (Fig. 1.32)	Salicylates, antibiotics, morphine
Erythema multiforme (Fig. 1.12)	Sulphonamides, penicillins, (including Stevens–Johnson variant) phenylbutazone, barbiturates.
Erythroderma (Fig. 1.6)	Allopurinol, gold, isoniazid, phenylbutazone
Toxic epidermal necrolysis (Fig. 8.46)	Barbiturates, phenytoin, penicillin, phenylbutazone
Allergic vasculitis (Fig. 1.41 and 1.42)	Sulphonamides, thiazides, phenylbutazone
Purpura (Fig. 1.36)	Sulphonamides, thiazides, quinine, phenylbutazone
Lichenoid eruptions (Figs. 8.47 and 5.16)	Antimalarials, non-steroidal anti-inflammatory drugs, gold, phenothiazines
Psoriasis	Exacerbated by antimalarials, lithium, beta-blockers
Acneiform eruptions (Fig. 5.28)	Lithium, oral contraceptives, androgenic and glucocorticoid steroids, anticonvulsant and antituberculous drugs
Fixed drug eruption (Fig. 1.116, 6.11 and 4.89)	Tetracyclines, sulphonamides, quinine, barbiturates, paracetamol

Table 3
Drug Eruptions and their Causes *(continued)*

Reaction Pattern	Drugs which Commonly Cause Reaction
Photosensitivity (Fig. 8.13 and 8.14)	Thiazides, sulphonamides, phenothiazines, quinine, tetracyclines
Pigmentation (Fig. 6.17 and 6.18)	Oral contraceptives, phenothiazines, amiodarone, antimalarial drugs
Hair loss (Fig. 4.7)	Cytotoxic agents, anticoagulants, antithyroid drugs, oral contraceptives, retinoids
Hypertrichosis	Minoxidil, cyclosporin, diazoxide

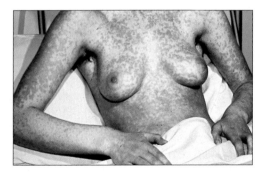

Fig. 8.45 Drug eruption
This explosive, symmetrical and maculo-papular rash appeared two days after starting ampicillin for a sore throat. Infectious mononucleosis was subsequently diagnosed but ampicillin reactions also occur frequently with cytomegalovirus infections and lymphatic leukaemia.

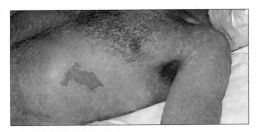

Fig. 8.46 Toxic epidermal necrolysis
A severe reaction, in this case to indomethacin. The patient had a generalized eruption. The raw area is where the epidermis is separating from the dermis. Nikolski's sign was positive.

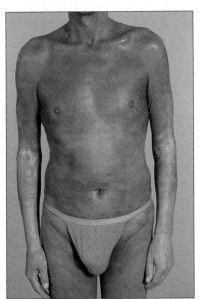

Fig. 8.47 Lichenoid drug eruption
An extensive lichenoid drug eruption, which eventually faded leaving striking hyperpigmentation.

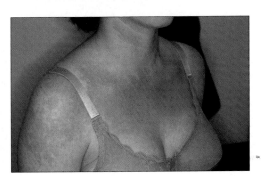

Fig. 8.48 Drug eruption
This striking erythema occurred at the same site, with monotonous regularity, at the beginning of menstruation. It was not due to a hormonal cause, as she and her general practitioner had thought, but to paracetamol taken for dysmenorrhoea.

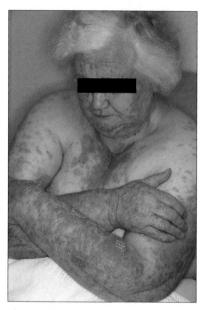

Fig. 8.49 Drug eruption
Striking eruption came up one week after starting chlorpropamide treatment. It disappeared on withdrawal of the drug.

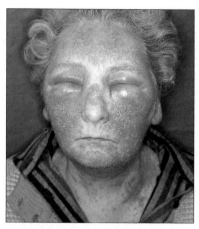

Fig. 8.50 Drug reaction
An acute eczematous reaction with erythema, weeping, crusting and marked periorbital oedema. The patient was apyrexial and did not feel ill. The culprit was a topical antihistamine. Reproduced with permission from Edwards, Bouchier, Haslett et al (eds), Davidson's Principles and Practice of Medicine, 17th edn., 1995, Churchill-Livingstone, Edinburgh.

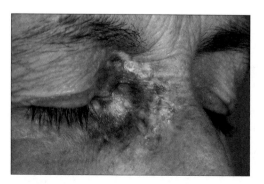

Fig. 8.51 Skin changes after radiotherapy
This typical mixture of atrophy, telangiectasia and patchy pigmentation marks the site where a small basal cell carcinoma had been treated with radiotherapy several years previously.

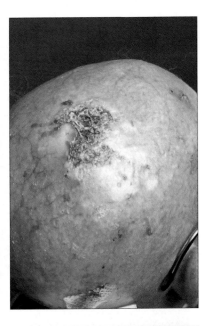

Fig. 8.52 Cutaneous atrophy following radiotherapy

At one time radiotherapy was considered a good treatment for scalp ringworm. This patient's thin but tightly bound down skin, and absence of hair, are late sequelae of this therapy. The area has been prone to develop keratoses and even squamous cell carcinomas.

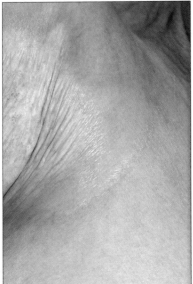

Fig. 8.53 Morphoea following radiotherapy

This classic plaque of morphoea developed in an area which had been irradiated two years previously. The patient and oncologist were reassured that it was not a local recurrence of the original tumour.

Chapter 9

Sensations

Some skin lesions can themselves generate unpleasant sensations such as pain or itch. In addition, some skin problems are secondary to neurological abnormalities. This chapter provides examples of each process.

ITCHING

Localized itching usually has an obvious skin cause; so, sometimes, has generalized itching. In every case a search has to be made for a treatable surface cause such as **atopic eczema** (Figs. 1.16, and 9.1), **lichen planus** (Figs. 5.12–5.15), **scabies** (Fig. 9.2), **lice** (Fig. 9.3 and 9.4) or **fibre glass**, accepting that diagnostic lesions may be hard to find. Only then should an internal cause be considered.

With a **lymphoma** (Fig. 9.5), itching may occur long before other manifestations; in contrast, when chronic **renal failure** is responsible for itching, the underlying cause is usually already well-known. Clues to other causes of itching include the stigmata of **hyperthyroidism** (Fig. 7.8), the jaundice and easy bruising of obstructive **liver disease** (Figs. 9.6 and 6.28), groups of small blisters in **dermatitis herpetiformis** (Figs. 1.107, 1.108 and 3.25) and the provocation of itching by a hot bath in **polycythaemia**. Itching, with or without a visible rash, is common in **pregnancy**.

The itching of **elderly people** may be due to inconspicuous dryness of the skin or asteatotic eczema (Figs. 7.4 and 7.5). **Psychogenic pruritus** (Fig. 9.7) does exist but should not be considered until organic causes have been excluded.

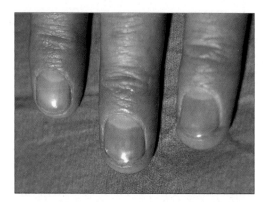

Fig. 9.1 Shiny nails
An important physical sign arising secondary to longterm rubbing and scratching of the skin. In this case the problem was atopic eczema.

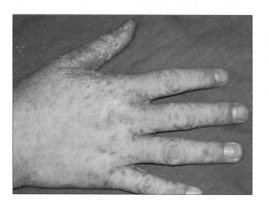

Fig. 9.2 Scabies
A chronic example, in which the burrows between the fingers and on the sides of the hand have become heavily eczematized.

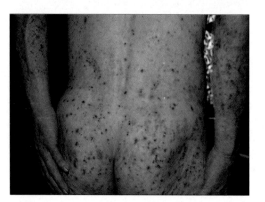

Fig. 9.3 Body Lice
Suspect this when itching occurs against a background of obvious self-neglect. Clothing should be examined for the presence of eggs in the inner seams.

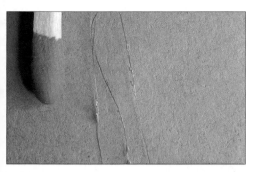

Fig. 9.4 Pubic lice
Tiny eggs (nits) are attached to these detached pubic hairs. The match head gives the scale.

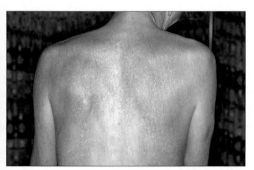

Fig. 9.5 Hodgkin's disease
This patient itched for two years before any trace of a lymphoma could be found. During this time her skin became increasingly pigmented, and many small white scars followed scratching. Note the spared area in the centre of the back which she could not reach.

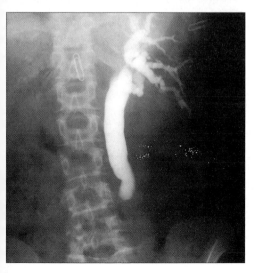

Fig. 9.6 Carcinoma of the ampulla of Vater
A tiny tumour here blocked the common bile duct causing severe itching but minimal jaundice.

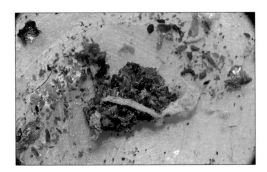

Fig. 9.7 Psychogenic pruritus
Parasitophobia — affected patients usually bring to the clinic a collection of 'specimens' such as these. Microscopy shows no parasites.

NUMBNESS

The combination of a defect in pain sensation plus trauma underlies the neurotrophic ulcers of **tabes dorsalis, spinal dysraphism, spinal cord injuries** and the **hereditary sensory neuropathies. Leprosy** and **diabetes** are the commonest causes (Figs. 9.8–9.11).

In **syringomyelia**, loss of sensation leads to repeated minor injuries and burns of the hands and arms. Most cases of the **trigeminal trophic syndrome** follow attempts to treat trigeminal neuralgia by surgery or alcohol injections. The resultant paraesthesiae make the patient keen to pick at the area so that a crescentic ulcer appears beside the nose (Fig. 9.12).

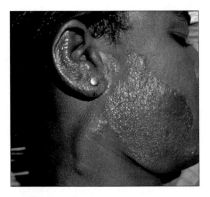

Fig. 9.8 Leprosy
The gross swelling of the nerve adjacent to this tuberculoid plaque was due to a type I LEPRA reaction to treatment. The plaque itself was already anaesthetic.

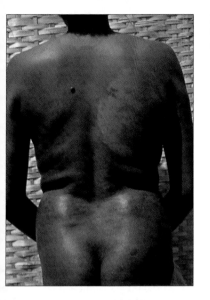

Fig. 9.9 Borderline leprosy
Large areas of hypopigmentation and
cutaneous anaesthesia.

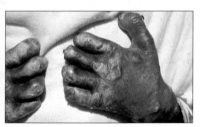

Fig. 9.10 Leprosy
Severe tissue destruction follows longterm
sensory loss in the hands.

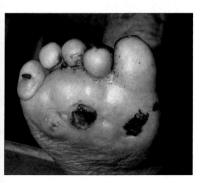

Fig. 9.11 Neuropathic ulcers
Microvascular disease and neuropathy
combine to cause these deep but painless
ulcers in a diabetic foot.

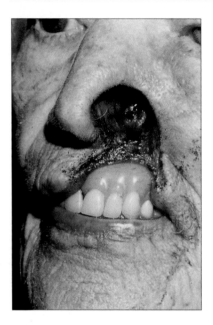

Fig. 9.12 Trigeminal trophic syndrome
An operation for trigeminal neuralgia, some 20 years before, was responsible for this. A curious type of paraesthesia, a sensation described as like a worm wriggling in the skin, lead to remorseless picking and an increasing loss of tissue.

PAIN

Pain is an unusual skin symptom and its presence may help in making a diagnosis.

PAINFUL TUMOURS

Neuroma and neurofibroma
Most common is a tender neuroma within a surgical scar.

Glomus tumour
Solitary lesions, most common on the extremities and under nails, are painful (Fig. 9.13). Multiple lesions tend to be asymptomatic.

Leiomyomas
These occur as groups of pink firm dermal nodules. Pain is provoked by changes in temperature, especially cooling, touching and emotional stress.

Angiolipoma
These resemble ordinary lipomas but are often painful and bluish rather than skin-coloured.

Corns and warts
Corns are common on the top of toe joints and under prominent metatarsals. Some **plantar warts** are painful too. They can be distinguished from corns by the tiny black dots or bleeding points seen when they are pared down (Fig. 9.14).

Painful piezogenic papules
These are herniations of fat on the side of the heel. They appear and hurt when weight is put on the heel (Fig. 9.15).

Subungual exostoses
These are often painful (Fig. 9.16).

PAINFUL INFLAMMATORY LESIONS

Cutaneous vasculitis
Vasculitis is painful whatever size of vessel is affected (Fig. 9.17). Painful, palpable purpura make up the classic triad of small vessel vasculitis (anaphylactoid purpura) (Fig. 1.41). Henoch-Schönlein purpura is a vasculitis of small vessels, usually of children, associated with arthritis and abdominal pain. The lesions of **erythema nodosum** (Fig. 1.14) may be exquisitely tender.

Herpes zoster
Pain occurs early, before erythema or blisters appear. In the elderly (Figs. 1.96 and 1.111), post-herpetic neuralgia may last for years.

Toxic epidermal necrolysis (Lyell's disease)
The skin becomes red and painful, and then peels off in sheets, like a scald (Fig. 8.46). This reaction is usually drug-induced, especially by sulphonamides, phenytoin, butazones and phenolphthalein. It may also occur in graft versus host disease, lymphoma and leukaemia, or after radiotherapy.

Chrondrodermatitis
These corn-like lesions are common on the side of the ear (Fig. 9.18). Inflammation of the underlying cartilage causes enough pain on pressure to wake sufferers repeatedly at night.

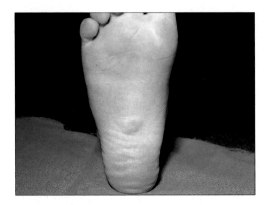

Fig. 9.13 Glomus tumour
This purplish nodule was painful enough to make walking difficult. Under the nails, much smaller lesions can cause exquisite pain.

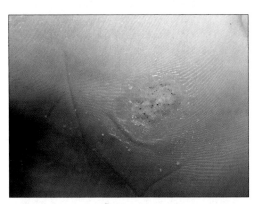

Fig. 9.14 A pared wart
Many thrombosed capillaries show up as small black dots — corns do not have these.

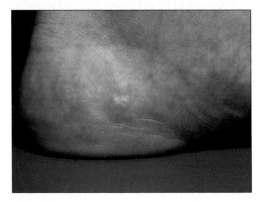

Fig. 9.15 Painful piezogenic papules
Herniations of fat on the side of the heel become prominent on standing and are then painful.

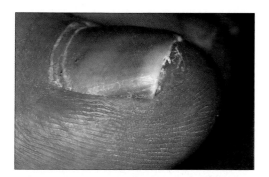

Fig. 9.16 Subungual exostosis

An exostosis arising from the terminal phalanyx has grown up under the free border of the nail and hurts when touched or pressed on by shoes.

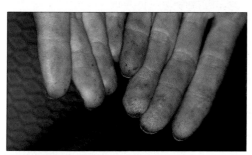

Fig. 9.17 Systemic lupus erythematosus

The small finger tip infarcts were very painful.

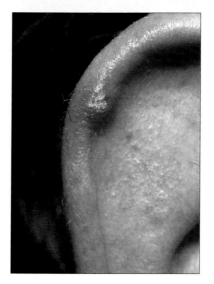

Fig. 9.18 Chondrodermatitis nodularis helicis chronica

A less clumsy name is painful nodule of the ear. These are common corn-like protuberances on the outer aspect of the rim of the ear. They combine inflammation of the skin and of the underlying cartilage. Lesions are benign but so painful that turning onto the ear at night will wake the patient up repeatedly.

ODOUR

Body odour is partly due to the bacterial decomposition of apocrine sweat. It is accentuated by lack of washing and by the overgrowth of commensal axillary organisms, as in trichomycosis axillaris (Fig. 9.19). A strong aroma also follows the digestion of keratin by commensal diphtheroids when sweaty feet are enclosed in occlusive shoes. **Pitted keratolysis** is the term used for the moth-eaten appearance of the soles which accompanies this (Fig. 7.7). Bacteria are also responsible for the smell of infected ulcers and ulcerated tumours; the odour of decay may be a clue to apical sepsis when a dental sinus drains outwards through the facial skin (Fig. 1.134). In the rare '**fish odour syndrome**', trimethylamine in the urine, sweat and breath causes the characteristic smell.

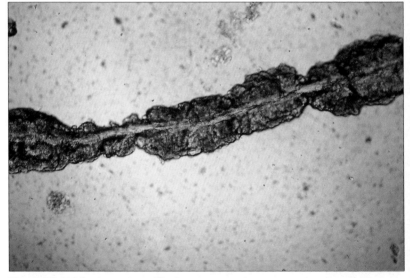

Fig. 9.19 Trichomycosis axillaris
Even in normal people the axillary hairs may be coated with an overgrowth of diphtheroid organisms, usually appearing yellow. These hairs fluoresce brightly under Wood's light.

Chapter 10

Timings

PRESENT AT BIRTH

Port wine stains usually affect the face (Fig. 3.12). Complications include glaucoma and the Sturge–Weber syndrome in which an accompanying vascular malformation of the meninges causes epilepsy and mental retardation. In the **Klippel–Trenaunay–Weber syndrome** (Fig. 10.1), port wine stains on a limb, usually present from birth, are associated with soft tissue and sometimes with bony hypertrophy.

Strictly speaking, **strawberry naevi** (capillary-cavernous haemangiomas) appear in the first few days of life rather than at birth (Fig. 10.2). Unusually large or multiple lesions may sequester platelets and cause bleeding (the **Kasabach–Merritt syndrome**). A **naevus anaemicus** (Fig. 6.25) is an irregular area of skin pallor sometimes seen in neurofibromatosis which does not become red after rubbing.

Epidermal naevi may be small and single (Fig.2.35), or extensive and multiple (Figs. 2.34 and 2.36) following Blaschko's lines. Sebaceous differentiation is common on the head and neck (naevus sebaceus) (Figs. 10.3 and 5.57). **Congenital melanocytic naevi** (Fig. 6.9) are common, usually small, and an isolated abnormality, though giant ones also occur (Fig. 1.57). Lesions on the lower back may be associated with spina bifida (Fig. 4.13). **Connective tissue naevi** (Fig. 7.15) may be present at birth or develop later. The shagreen patches of **tuberous sclerosis** (Fig. 10.4) are soft, raised skin-coloured lesions over the lower back. The rather yellower lesions of **juvenile elastoma** are one component of the Buschke-Ollendorf syndrome; osteopoikilosis (multiple areas of opacity in long bones (Fig. 7.16)) is the other.

Important **genodermatoses** present at birth include incontinentia pigmenti (Fig. 10.5), aplasia cutis, the various types of epidermolysis bullosa, the Harlequin foetus (Fig. 10.6) and the collodion baby (Fig. 10.7).

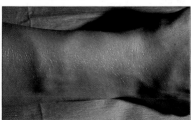

Fig. 10.1 Klippel–Trenaunay--Weber syndrome
This limb contained multiple small arterio-venous shunts. It was bigger than the other arm, hotter, more hairy and had an obvious varicose vein. The associated capillary naevus was faint and not shown here.

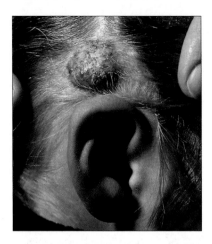

Fig. 10.2 Strawberry naevus
Increasing surface pallor suggests that this one is already undergoing involution.

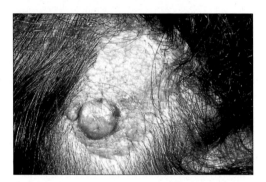

Fig. 10.3 Naevus sebaceus
A single naevus sebaceus, present as a yellow hairless area from birth, became slightly raised at puberty. During adult life tumours may develop upon it, such as the basal cell carcinoma seen here.

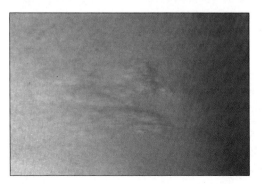

Fig. 10.4 Connective tissue naevi
These are an important part of tuberous sclerosis. Juvenile elastomas look rather similar and are associated with osteopoikilosis.

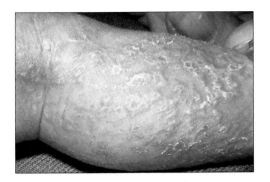

Fig. 10.5 Incontinentia pigmenti
Lines and groups of vesico-pustules are present at birth. This is an X-linked dominant condition, usually lethal before birth in males.

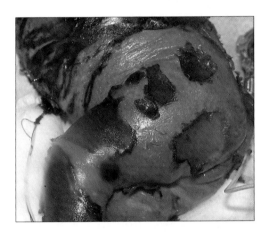

Fig. 10. 6 Harlequin foetus
The hard, keratotic, roughly diamond-shaped plates are separated by glistening pink skin to produce a pattern faintly reminiscent of the traditional harlequin costume. These babies seldom survive.

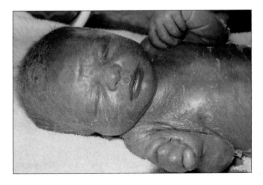

Fig 10.7 Collodion baby
The skin is tight and looks as if it has been covered with cellophane. This layer is shed within a few days. Usually the forerunner of severe ichthyosis.

ADOLESCENCE

At this age, personal appearance has become important and many skin abnormalities, present since birth, are shown to doctors. In addition, an increase in sebum production leads to greasy hair and skin, and in apocrine secretions to body odour. Excessive sweating on the palms and soles is common but seldom of medical significance.

Acne vulgaris (Figs. 5.20 and 5.21)usually starts in the mid-teens and resolves by the mid-twenties, although it persists to the age of 40 in 5% of women and 1% of men. Acne is also a feature of the polycystic ovary, adrenogenital and Cushing's syndromes.

Premature puberty occurs in conditions such as the McCune–Albright syndrome (Fig. 6.4), tuberous sclerosis, neurofibromatosis (Figs. 6.2, 6.3 and 3.23), Cushing's syndrome, adrenal tumours, congenital adrenal hyperplasia, ovarian and testicular tumours. **Delayed puberty** also has many causes. Look for associated signs, such as the obesity, short stature and mental retardation of the Prader-Willi syndrome and for the tall male with gynaecomastia of Klinefelter's syndrome.

PREGNANCY

Pigmentation gradually increases, particularly on the areolae and genital skin. More specific pigmentation occurs along the mid-line of the lower abdomen (the 'linea nigra') and on the face ('chloasma') (Fig. 6.13). As pregnancy proceeds, red **stretch marks** may appear (Fig. 10.8); these fade in the puerperium but leave permanent silvery linear defects. **Vascular changes** during pregnancy include spider naevi (Fig. 1.30), palmar erythema (Fig. 1.1), varicose veins and haemorrhoids, deep venous thrombosis and gingival epulis. The **polymorphic eruption of pregnancy** (Fig. 10.9) is not uncommon.

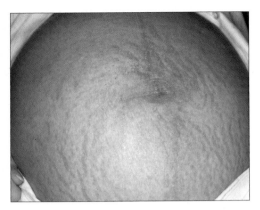

Fig. 10.8 Stretch marks
These are common in
pregnancy.

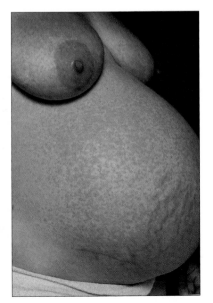

**Fig. 10.9 Polymorphic eruption of
pregnancy (sometimes also
known as PUPPP which stands for
pruritic urticarial papules and
plaques of pregnancy)**
This itchy eruption begins in the last trimester
of pregnancy and consists of urticated
lesions often most striking on the stretch
marks. Seldom associated with foetal
morbidity, and clears soon after childbirth.

227

MIDDLE AGE

There are few signs specific to middle age. Any changes are the start of those seen in old age. **Flushing** (Fig. 8.1) is common at the menopause. The term **keratoderma climactericum** describes the hard skin on the palms and soles, especially round the heels, seen in a few menopausal women (Fig. 10.10).

A **diagonal crease across the ear lobes** (Fig. 10.11) is thought by some to be associated with a liability to hypertension and diabetes.

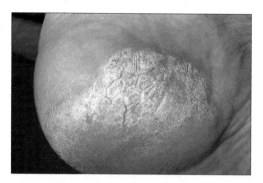

Fig. 10.10 Post-menopausal keratoderma
This thick hyperkeratosis appears on the palms and soles. Some consider it to be a response to hormonal changes, as it often occurs in middle-aged women at the menopause.

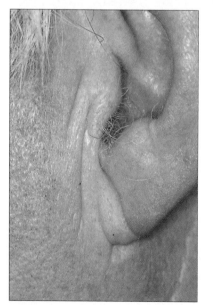

Fig. 10.11 Diagonal ear-lobe crease
A dubious sign of a predisposition to diabetes or hypertension.

OLD AGE

Ultraviolet radiation (UVR) is the main cause of ageing of white skin. Prolonged exposure damages elastic fibres and this leads to a yellow, pebbly appearance **(elastosis)** (Fig. 8.24), most noticeable on the back of the neck and the temples. **Senile comedones** (Fig. 10.12) may also appear, often around the eyes. The skin sags and wrinkles once the dermis has lost its elastic recoil (Fig 10.13).

Some rare syndromes accelerate ageing, both of the skin and of internal organs. **Werner's syndrome** is an autosomal recessive trait; patients are small and prematurely grey haired (Fig. 4.15). Persistent ulcers appear (Fig. 10.14) especially over the protruding metatarsal heads (Fig. 10.15). Diabetes is an early complication and bilateral cataracts develop in the twenties. Premature arteriosclerosis usually causes death before the age of 50 and there is also a high incidence of systemic malignancy.

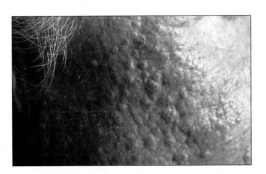

Fig. 10.12 Senile comedones
A striking example of a common abnormality.

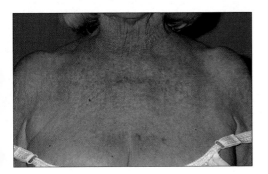

Fig. 10.13 Skin ageing
The contrast is obvious between the wrinkled blotchy exposed areas and the rest of the skin.

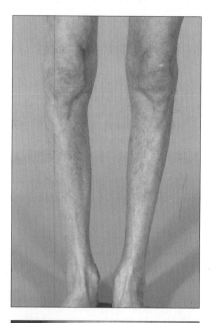

Fig. 10.14 Werner's syndrome
The thin spindly legs of a sufferer aged 26.

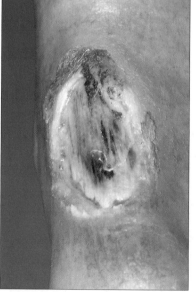

Fig. 10.15 Werner's syndrome
A deep ulcer above the heel — down to the Achilles tendon.

Index

Note: numbers refer to page numbers, not figure numbers

antihistamines 210
antimalarial drugs 127, 208
antiphospolipid antibody syndrome 77
anxiety state 166
Apert's syndrome 135, 138
aphthous ulcers 106, 109
aplasia cutis 223
argyria 115, 120
arsenical keratoses 143, 148
arthritis mutilans 129
asteatosis 163, 165
ataxia telangiectasia 13, 102
atopic eczema 49
  eczema herpeticum 91
  itching 213, 214
  keratoconus 102
  lichenification 169
  post-inflammatory hyperpigmentation 150
  umbilicated lesions 80
atrophie blanche 37, 38
atypical mole syndrome 150, 153

bacteria
  odour 222
  pustules 51, 54
bacterial endocarditis 115, 119
bacterial folliculitis 85
bacterial infection, perianal 122
bacterial toxaemia 1
balanitis, circinate 122, 125
barbiturates 50
basal cell carcinoma 26, 29–30, 37, 41, 62
  cicatricial 93
  eyelids 101, 104
  scalp 100
  scars 187, 189
  sebaceous naevus 148, 224
Beau's lines 114, 117
Becker's naevus 94, 98
Behçet's disease 102, 106, 109
  genital ulcers 122, 125
  trauma 197
Berloque dermatitis 70, 193
beta-blockers
  lichenoid eruptions 132, 134
  psoriasis/psoriasiform eruption 127

Blaschko's lines 70, 74, 75, 143, 149
  epidermal naevi 223
blisters 44–50
blood dyscrasias 37
blood vessel damage 18, 20
body odour 222
Borrelia burgdorferi 61
Bowen's disease
  psoriasiform lesions 127
  warty 143, 146
brachyonychia 115
branchial cysts 55
branchial sinus 58
breast tumours 26, 35
bronchiectasis 115, 120
Brunsting—Perry type of pemphigoid 101
bullous dermatosis, chronic 68
bullous disorders
  scalp 100
  urticarial 139
bullous impetigo, blisters 45
burn scarring 93, 95, 187
Buschke—Ollendorf syndrome 168, 170, 223
busulphan 150
butterfly eruptions 68–9

C1 esterase inhibitor deficiency 16, 17
café au lait patches 149, 151
calcinosis 171, 172
  circumscripta 184
calcium deposits 181, 184
Campbell de Morgan spots 21, 22, 26
Candida albicans 122
candidal intertrigo 83
candidiasis, oral 106, 108
capillaritis, benign 150
capillary malformations 87, 102
carbuncle 93
carcinoid, flushing attacks 14, 185, 186
carcinoma
  of ampulla of Vater 215
  metastatic 93, 95
  telangiectoides 35
carcinomatosis, calcium deposits 181
carotenaemia 160, 161
cellulitis, dissecting of scalp 135